MW01129580

*„I love this book. It's not just that Michio ...
who has real experience in day-to-day mo ...
as taught macrobiotics to large numbers ...
ses what macrobiotics is and how to brinç ...*
**Mayumi Niimi, Madonna's private macrobiotic chef;
author of Mayumi's Kitchen: Macrobiotic Cooking for Body and Soul.**

*„The Macrobiotic Kitchen in Ten Easy Steps is the definitive guide to healthful eating.
Engaging and clearly written, it shows step by step how to transition to a new way of
thinking about food. It will change your life.“*
**Neal D. Barnard, MD, president, Physicians Committee for Responsible Medicine;
adjunct associate professor of medicine,
George Washington University School of Medicine, Washington, DC**

*„The Macrobiotic Kitchen in Ten Easy Steps is beautiful, thorough, and immensely practi-
cal—all at once. Having practiced macrobiotics for many decades, Gabriele possesses precious wisdom and wonderful recipes that harmonize well with Michio Kushi's macrobiotic
teachings. This book belongs in every healthy kitchen.“*
Jessica Porter, author of The MILF Diet and The Hip Chick's Guide to Macrobiotics.

*„With this book in collaboration with her father-in-law, Michio Kushi, Gabriele Kushi
offers her unique recipes and macrobiotic wisdom to all of us who want to live a healthful
life.“*
Sandy Pukel, owner of Holistic Holiday at Sea

*"I can't imagine two people more qualified to write **The Macrobiotic Kitchen in Ten
Easy Steps** than Michio and Gabriele Kushi. Michio is the master teacher who brought
macrobiotics to the West more than 40 years ago. He has been lecturing and consulting
ever since. Gabriele, his daughter-in-law, brings a global perspective and timeless aesthetic
that is truly unique. Together they cook up a beautiful, healthy cuisine. Bon appetit!"*
Eric Utne, founder, Utne Reader

*„Merely imbibing the photographs in this delicious book is superb nourishment! Here is a
simple, beautiful, nourishing, step-by-step guide to freedom from drugs and disease with
a dietary plan that heals you and the environment at the same time. Who better than
Gabriele Kushi and her father-in-law Michio Kushi to guide us on the journey of discovery
on the river of yin/yang? The macrobiotic tenet—`Eat what is in season where you live`—is
one of the easiest to follow, and one of the most potent, food guidelines ever articulated.
`Macrobiotics` means `long life`, and that says it all. If you're interested in a long, healthy,
creative, enjoyable life, you need this book."*
Susun Weed, author of the Wise Woman Herbal Series

*„The Macrobiotic Kitchen in Ten Easy Steps by Gabriele Kushi and Michio Kushi is a fun-
damental book to anyone who wishes to start a macrobiotic or vegetarian diet or simply
start to eat in a more conscious way. Actually, even people who have been macrobiotic
or vegetarian for a long time will have a lot to learn from this wonderful book. In its over
200 pages, the authors will guide you through all the steps necessary to master the kitchen, from your posture and attitude when you cook to how to choose healthy ingredients
for a balanced menu. In all my years of practice I have seen many cookbooks and this is
without any doubt one of the more complete and clear you can find. You can't miss it.“*
Francisco Varatojo, Macrobiotic Institute of Portugal

Dedication

*This book is dedicated
to the Seven Generations
who come after us.*

The Macrobiotic Kitchen in Ten Easy Steps

— Balanced Eating in the 21ˢᵗ Century —

Gabriele Kushi

With Michio Kushi

Foreword by Neal D. Barnard, MD

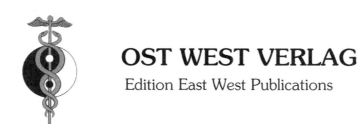

OST WEST VERLAG

Edition East West Publications

Title: The Macrobiotic Kitchen in Ten Easy Steps
          – Balanced Eating in the 21ˢᵗ Century –
by Gabriele Kushi with Michio Kushi
© Gabriele Kushi
First published by Ost West Verlag, Voelklingen, Germany, 2015
Edition East West Publications
Consulting Editor: Richard Theobald

All food photography by Allen Brown
Portrait of Michio Kushi courtesy of Michio Kushi
Portrait Photo of Gabriele Kushi: Noah Wolf

Bibliographic information of the German National Library:
This publication is listed in the Catalogue of the German National Library.
Data are available at http://d-nb.info/1076585922
ISBN 978-3-930564-40-8

The material in this book is intended to provide information on natural and whole foods from a
macrobiotic, one peaceful world point of view. The views expressed and options presented in this book
on any foods, therapies, or remedies are for informational purposes only, and are not intended as medical
or nutritional advice, research material, or prescriptions for treatment for any condition. For detailed
guidance on dietary change, consult a medical doctor, a nutritionist, and/or a qualified macrobiotic
counselor. Neither the publisher nor the authors can take responsibility for your specific health or allergy
needs that may require medical supervision or for any adverse reactions to the recipes contained in this
book.

Internet addresses given in this book were accurate at the time it went to press.

Table of Contents

Foreword

In our research at the Physicians Committee for Responsible Medicine in Washington, DC, we have seen the power that carefully prepared foods can have. People with weight problems, heart disease, diabetes, and chronic pain come through our doors and make diet changes in hopes of improving their health. The results are quick and often surprising: excess weight melts away, heart disease and diabetes begin to reverse, and chronic pain vanishes. Everyone gets their own result, of course, but overall we have found that a change in diet is much more powerful than anyone would have guessed—often more powerful than prescription medications.

When I was in medical school, nutrition was given only cursory attention; we were taught to rely on pharmaceuticals rather than to address the nutritional causes of medical conditions. I reached a turning point two decades ago at a symposium for physicians presented by Michio Kushi in Boston. Along with a team of physician instructors, he brought dietary information to a whole new level. Many of the concepts they discussed were totally new to me and to the other doctors attending the course, and I concentrated on their words with great intensity.

Many of the foods he and his team mentioned were new to me, too. Growing up in Fargo, North Dakota, I knew about roast beef, baked potatoes, and corn, but had never tasted brown rice or miso soup and wasn't so sure about broccoli or cucumbers, either. But I met several people who had tried the approach Michio described. They had put it to work and had achieved wonderful success.

And then I discovered something else. Eating macrobiotic meals over the course of a few days during the seminar, I felt terrific myself. Somehow, these foods just felt right. Tasty, nourishing, sometimes a bit adventurous—they were new, exciting, energizing, and obviously worked in perfect harmony with body chemistry.

Over the years, scientists have taken an interest in macrobiotics and have put it to the test in rigorous research studies. Concepts that had been described in terms of yin, yang, and balance are now studied using terms like statistical significance, P-values, and confidence intervals. And we now know that, indeed, this age-old healthful tradition has the power to heal.

This book puts all of this into your hands. Let me encourage you to try its step-by-step approach and to share what you learn with others in your life. I hope that you find, as we have, that carefully prepared foods are as delightful for the taste buds as they are powerful for health.

Neal D. Barnard, MD
President, Physicians Committee for Responsible Medicine, Adjunct Associate Professor of Medicine, George Washington University School of Medicine, Washington, DC

About the Book

The food you eat creates your cells and supports your life. In addition, the elements of your whole lifestyle, including your environment, your thoughts, your emotions, and your actions, sustain you. When you choose a *nourishing* lifestyle and bring *awareness* to your food habits, you bring an abundance of satisfaction and good health into your life. Small adjustments here and there go a long way toward realizing life-giving abundance.

It's too easy these days to just grab a bite and not cook at home, *even if you have been introduced to macrobiotics or another healthy way of eating in the past.* As a result, your energy can become chaotic and not strong enough to carry you through the day. If you're like most people, you struggle with cutting down or eliminating fast foods, or you may eat snacks all day, with no good meals for days. Made-from-scratch home cooking rarely happens, and many meals are replaced by packaged, refined foods (often disguised as "natural" foods) loaded with sugar, salt, hydrogenated fats, and chemicals. If these sound like your eating habits, ask yourself: *Am I at risk for ending up with a major health concern? Am I ready to make a change that might save my life?*

Changing to healthier eating habits is on a lot of people's minds these days. Slimming diets, mega dose supplements, and protein powders are promoted as ways to help, but too often they become replacements for the basics of healthy eating. Advertisements even endorse supersized and fake foods as acceptable in a good diet. These different approaches can boggle your mind. It can be hard to know where to start and what to do.

Other lifestyle habits also affect your health. An overly busy schedule can lead to burnout. You may use too many electronic gadgets every day at work and then late in the evening and on weekends. This may lead to sleepless nights. City life and long stressful commutes keep you from spending reinvigorating time outside in fresh air. You may be yearning to eat a good quality meal and to be in nature among the trees or out walking in a green meadow. Where can you begin to follow these instincts? How do you get yourself out of this daily rut?

You know that today's lifestyles and eating habits have a shadow side. Many sicknesses begin when you get away from nature and don't eat healthy, life-supporting foods. Health organizations have confirmed this negative relationship for decades. Scientific research has shown that the lifestyles we lead and the foods we eat influence our health, and our own experiences confirm it. Almost daily, we hear that close friends, family members, neighbors, or people at work are diagnosed with cancer, are overweight, have diabetes, MS, or heart disease... and the list goes on. Maybe you fall into one of these categories yourself or have thought, what next? Is this the flip side of modern living?

In the end, it's up to you to protect and maintain your health. Why not start doing the very best to take care of your body right now? Ask yourself: What do I have the most influence on and control over? What can I actually change, starting today? Isn't it the food you put into your mouth?

This book will support you, *Step by healthful Step,* to a fresh start and a renewed resolve to choose natural, whole foods and sound lifestyle strategies. The macrobiotic approach to living, balancing yin and yang and eating in harmony with nature, provides the framework for a health-supportive lifestyle. The natural foods recipes will assist you in making the shift to healthy, seasonal eating without stress.

The kitchen fire is the center of your home and your life—the base for a healthy lifestyle. Healthy eating habits are important in order to create and manifest your dreams. You receive the most nourishment for yourself and your loved ones when you embrace balancing principles in your kitchen and eat your own cooked food. And eating out can still be a harmonious and joyful experience when you know how to choose the right foods for these occasions.

You can begin today. How? It's easy! Do it by gradually substituting healthy foods for less healthy ones, thus shifting your food habits naturally. Very few people can or should make a radical overnight transition from a diet of primarily meat and sugar to a plant-based diet that includes grains, beans, seeds, nuts, and vegetables. We believe that the best transition to macrobiotic natural foods and a balanced seasonal lifestyle is a slow-but-sure one, and that is why we wrote this book. Your body will have an easier time adjusting to the many new foods and preparation methods, and the gentle transition will be long lasting. Of course, if you want, you can also transform your eating habits more quickly if your life situation calls for it.

If you use the step-by-step approach, we suggest that you experiment with each Step for a two-week period. Study everything carefully, including the macrobiotic yin-yang information and seasonal food charts, and try out the recipes.

Start freshening up your lifestyle by eating green leafy vegetables during Step 1, and bring plants with large green leaves into your living areas, as these provide good oxygen. Learn all about why eating greens is important and the history of these wonderful foods.

Then continue to Step 2, with the whole grain food group, and incorporate the knowledge you gained in Step 1. Some people have a variety of allergic reactions to foods that contain gluten, as well as to soy, citrus, peanuts, dairy, and so forth, and sensitivities to chemicals in the food and the air. For your convenience, we provide gluten advice and suggest gluten-free grain replacements. Gluten-containing grains and foods are generally not bad foods if whole, natural and GMO free. Yet people with gluten sensitivities, allergies, or autoimmune sensitivities from various causes (for instance, overconsumption of refined and denatured gluten-containing flour products and white sugar) should avoid them.

As you move through each Step, you will slowly and easily have all the food groups, recipes, and lifestyle changes under your belt, and you will have created a wellness kitchen for a lifetime. By using the methods in this book, you can leave difficult circumstances and unhealthful patterns behind and move closer to realizing your dreams. Many positive things will happen, and they will unfold naturally.

Gabriele Kushi and Michio Kushi

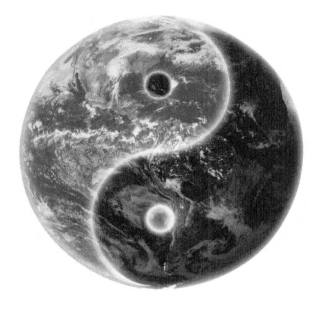

The Art and Science of Macrobiotics

Macrobiotics (Greek: large or long life) embraces the art and science of living sustainably and eating in harmony with the rhythm of the seasons to further nature's healing forces for personal and planetary health and peace.

The macrobiotic teachings offer a relearning process for the common sense and wisdom of natural ways that have often been forgotten or overlooked. Millions of people on this planet are actively practicing a macrobiotic way of life because it makes them feel good and they want to support a sustainable and peaceful future. Connecting with the seasonal changes by using the foods that grow locally and balancing them with your personal needs and goals will open your connections with nature. Take the first Step, and the rest will follow with ease. Your intuition will sharpen, and you will notice changes that take place within yourself.

Macrobiotics Influence in the World

Throughout history, philosophers and physicians often used the term *macrobiotic* to promote well being and longevity, and the diet has been practiced widely throughout history by all major civilizations and cultures. The earliest recorded use of the term is in the writings of Hippocrates. The nineteenth-century German physician Christoph Wilhelm Hufeland published the first book with macrobiotics in the title.[1] Hufeland advocated a moderate style of living, although he did not incorporate the concept of yin and yang balance and its applications that we know as macrobiotics today.

Founder of the twentieth-century macrobiotic movement, the late George Ohsawa from Japan, drew on the Eastern philosophy of yin and yang, studied the work of Eastern scholars, and applied traditional Japanese food and medicinal approaches to develop the modern foundation of macrobiotic teachings. Through extensive travels, numerous books, and his Ignoramus School in Japan, he, along with his wife Lima and his students Michio and Aveline Kushi (among others) brought the macrobiotic teachings to the world after World War II to further a peaceful, sustainable approach to life.[2]

Beginning in the 1950s, macrobiotic educators have developed a vast library of literature [3][4][5] and established macrobiotic teaching facilities and food companies around the world. For instance, the late Aveline Kushi [6] devoted her life to making whole food products available by inspiring farmers to grow foods such as brown rice. The Kushis also opened the first macrobiotic natural foods store and distribution company in the US, Erewhon, in 1966. In Europe in 1957, Pierre Gevaert founded the first macrobiotic natural foods distribution and production company, named Lima in honor of George Ohsawa's wife.

Macrobiotics, with its many associate teachers and students around the world, opened the door for Eastern medicine and ways of life, and introduced profound thinking about nutrition and food as preventive and healing modalities. It acted as a catalyst for the acceptance of alternative and complementary medicine when the Kushi Institute, the premier center for macrobiotic learning, opened in the late 1970s in the United States and England, followed by branches in the Netherlands and Japan. In 1999, the Smithsonian Institution recognized Aveline and Michio Kushi's[7] contributions to the evolution of modern society when it archived documents and artifacts related to their macrobiotic work and established the *Michio and Aveline Kushi Collection, 1960-1997* at the National Museum of American History.

Prominent figures like Madonna, Gwyneth Paltrow, and actor and author Dirk Benedict[8] embrace the nourishing macrobiotic lifestyle. The late John Lennon, John Denver, Gloria Swanson, and author William Dufty[9] are all known to have practiced the art of macrobiotics.

Macrobiotic Health Benefits

The macrobiotic way of eating and lifestyle has helped to familiarize the world with the concepts of whole and natural foods. Western science has demonstrated the health-promoting benefits of the nutrients found in the natural foods used in a macrobiotic lifestyle. They are helpful for a strong immune system, reduction of high cholesterol levels, heart disease prevention, weight management, easing menopausal symptoms, and protecting against degenerative disease and cancer.[10] Medical professionals often refer their clients to macrobiotics for additional management of certain illnesses. Thus the macrobiotic way of life may be seen as beneficial during times of increasing cancer rates, heart disease, obesity, allergies, AIDS, and the hazards of environmental pollution, all conditions considered to be a result of imbalanced modern behaviors.

Articles on macrobiotic dietary and lifestyle benefits have been published in numerous scientific and medical journals. In 2000, an important study[11] of alternative treatments used by cancer patients reported that many such treatments, including a macrobiotic healing diet, are effective in reducing stress, minimizing discomfort, and giving patients a sense of control. Many people have also given testimonials about how they healed breast cancer, Crohn's disease, and other illnesses with a macrobiotic healing diet especially designed for them. Cases of major recoveries have been published in book form[12 13 14 15 16], with varying degrees of medical documentation.

The *macrobiotic healing diet*[17] is a specific nutritional and lifestyle program that is individually designed by a macrobiotic-certified counselor for people with a particular disease. It is a transitional and health-supportive plan that is adjusted during the course of recovery and then followed with the wider, *standard macrobiotic diet and lifestyle* approach. (For treatment and guidance in dietary change when you have a health condition, consult a medical doctor, a nutritionist, and/or a qualified macrobiotic counselor.)

The macrobiotic diet includes many food groups that other regimens overlook, and provides a yin-yang and seasonal approach that is centered on a balanced plant-based lifestyle. As macrobiotic theory says, everything is constantly changing, and so will your nourishment needs change with the season and over the years as you continue to practice good eating habits. Thus, eating animal foods, for instance, is an individual choice. The proportions of a standard macrobiotic diet can be adjusted according to your gender, age, cultural heritage, level of activity, personal needs, and health concerns, and the climate and environment you live in. Macrobiotics also embraces various lifestyle modalities like shiatsu, Do-In[18] (a form of self-massage), visualization, meditation, yoga, and outdoor activities like gardening, walks, or other activities that support and strengthen your body, mind, and spirit.

Macrobiotic Yin-Yang Principles

Macrobiotics integrates 5,000-year-old Eastern wisdom and modern Western science. The ancient philosophy of *yin-yang* provides the concepts and main principles macrobiotics embraces in its teachings. Yin, the expanding energy, and yang, the contracting energy, are the two fundamental, contrary, and complementary forces of nature. The macrobiotic application of yin and yang provides a practical and physical approach in all domains. It differs somewhat from the Traditional Chinese Medicine (TCM) teachings, which provide a more energetic and metaphysical viewpoint. Both systems use yin-yang; they just use it from a different point of view.

In macrobiotics, we use yin and yang to explain the unifying principles to balance influences in support of overall well being. We look at the diametrically opposed forces that are inherent in all things. You can see these ever-changing, contrasting, and balancing forces of nature at work in all existence, including our own lives. Examples include expansion and contraction, dark and bright, male and female, night and day, big and small, far and near, and hot and cold.

In your kitchen, observe the properties of vegetables that grow above the earth versus vegetables that grow under the earth, or of food that comes from colder climates versus warmer ones, and of refined food versus unrefined food. You can see it, for instance, in the different shapes—round and long, or the red and white colors of foods. There are yin-yang contrasts in how to cut your vegetables, such as big chunks or small matchsticks, and in the ways to cook food, such as steaming or pressure-cooking.

The seasonal use of various cooking methods and vegetables, when looked at from a yin and yang point of view, begins to make a lot of sense. The expanding (yin) and contracting (yang) concepts help you to balance your recipes to prepare sustainable, healthy meals. Certain foods are better to eat in the summer, like soft, watery summer squashes, and others support your energy during the winter, like hard winter squashes. The macrobiotic art and science of balancing the many different wonderful things in your life may give you some trials, yet when you grasp the idea, you can easily apply what you learn to all spheres of life. Start to apply your new knowledge in your kitchen by using the foods that grow in the season and climate zone you are in. Gradually, over time, as you follow nature's movements, your physical, mental, and emotional well-being will thank you for it.

A Balanced and Seasonal Way of Life

In macrobiotics you learn to reconnect to nature and observe the seasonal cycles and the use of whole foods to help you balance your daily life and health. Just as you choose your clothing according to the season, you can fine-tune your kitchen in harmony with seasonal vegetables, beans, and grains. In the spring, emphasize fresh foods and shorter cooking times. For example, when everything is sprouting, choose sprouted foods often, and if available, eat wild salads made with dandelion. In winter,

Examples of the contrasting and complementary Yin and Yang tendencies in nature		
	YIN	YANG
Function	Diffusion	Contraction
	Dispersion	Fusion
	Separation	Gathering
	Decomposition	Organisation
Movement	More inactive, slower	More activ, faster
Vibration	Shorter wave and higher	Longer wave and and lower
Direction	Ascent and vertical	Descent and horizontal
Position	More outward and peripheral	More inward and central
Weight	Lighter	Heavier
Temperature	Colder	Hotter
Light	Darker	Brighter
Humidity	More wet	More dry
Density	Thinner	Thicker
Size	Larger	Smaller
Shape	More expansive and fragile	More contractive and harder
Form	Longer	Shorter
Texture	Softer	Harder
Atomic particle	Elektron	Proton
Elements	N, O, K, Ca. etc.	H, C, Na, As, Mg. etc.
Environment	Vibration............Air............Water..............Earth	
Climatic effects	Tropical climate	Colder climate
Biological	More vegetable quality	M0re animal quality
Sex	Female	Male
Organ structure	More hollow and expansive	More compacted and condensed
Nerves	More peripheral, orthosympathetic	more central, parasympathetic
Attitude, emotion	More gentle, defensive	More active, aggresive
Work	More psychological and mental	More physical and social
Dimension	Space	Time

implement longer cooking styles and prepare hearty stews. By harmonizing your energy with the environment in this way, you are strengthening your body, mind, and spirit.

Examples of characteristic tendencies of Yin und Yang in foods and plants		
	YIN	**YANG**
Chemical components	More K and other yin- elements Less Na and other yang-elements	Less K and other yin-elements More Na and other yang-elements
Climatic influence	Grows more in warmer climate	Grows more in colder climate
Growing speed	Faster	Slower
Size	Larger, more expanded	Smaller, more compact
Height	Longer	Shorter
Water content	More juicy and watery	More dry
Texture	Softer	Harder
Growing direction	Vertically growing upward; expanding horizontally underground	Vertically growing downward; expanding horizontally above the ground
Leave sizes	Larger	Smaller
Leave edges	Smooth	Jagged
Cooking time	Shorter	Longer
Effect on the human organism after consumption	Chilling, relaxing, slowing down, calming, more need for sleep	Warming, stimulating, activating, exciting, less need for sleep
Nutritional components	Fat........protein........carbohydrate........mineral	
Taste	Spicy........sour........sweet........salty........bitter	
Odor	Stronger smell	Less smell

Spend time in nature such as wooded areas to balance indoor living. The more you do this, the better you will feel. Choose gardening, walking, running, biking, or other appropriate outdoor activities. Physical activity in natural environments seems to support mental health even better than indoor physical activity, according to experimental studies.[19] Observe nature, reflect, and be respectful of and grateful for everything, including your ancestors. Rejuvenate your body, mind, and spirit with appropriate weight bearing and stretching exercises, which provide the most benefits for a balanced lifestyle when done on a regular basis, either in natural or indoor environments. Spend relaxing time in meditation, do breathing exercises, and be mindful of your breath. Natural and harmonious living also calls for using natural fabrics in clothing and bedding, chemical-free household cleaning materials, sustainable gardening products, and organic cosmetics.

A balanced way of life supports organic, non-GMO natural agriculture and natural food processing and production. We raise environmental awareness while preserving a clean, natural environment and respecting animal life. We promote water conservation as well as natural technologies to purify and filter contaminated water, and a natural approach to physical and spiritual welfare.

Find opportunities to support these values. If possible, choose to work at a sustainable business, invest or shop at green companies, purchase green building materials, and work to preserve natural environments. Speak up against animal cruelty and shop for cruelty-free, non-animal-tested products. Live consciously and responsibly to leave a small footprint on this earth so that the Seven Generations who come after you have a place to live. This is also what Native American elders teach their young ones.

Natural, Whole Foods in Your Kitchen

Natural, whole foods contain strong nutrient and health-supportive properties that address your needs for a balanced, seasonal approach to cooking. Cook nutrient-dense whole foods without refined sugars and artificial sweeteners. Avoid processed foods, white flour, and foods containing chemical additives or hormones. Obtain quality spring or filtered chlorine-free water. Choose organic whenever possible, and avoid genetically modified (GMO) products. Be aware that products labeled "natural" might not be natural at all, as they could contain GMO or refined and chemically enhanced ingredients.

Create seasonally balanced meals with foods from the vast variety of the vegetable kingdom. Include whole grains, legumes (beans and tempeh), green leafy vegetables, root and round vegetables, raw foods, sea vegetables, seeds, nuts, fruits, herbs, unrefined oils, and sea salt. Create your menus with the freshest ingredients, and include a range of food groups to ensure adequate and balanced nutrition.

Thus the macrobiotic kitchen provides a nourishing, balanced, plant-based (vegan) baseline that can be modified and adjusted to your needs. Whether you choose to eat entirely vegan or opt to include some items from the animal kingdom, having a good knowledge about balanced eating habits is important. For non-vegan eating, we suggest first choosing ecologically harvested water animals like fish. Most fish digests easier then meat, plus fish often contains healthy fats. If you choose to eat from the land animal kingdom, choose animals that live free-range, are humanely raised, are fed organic, non-GMO, hormone-free, species-appropriate food, and are slaughtered ethically. In your macrobiotic kitchen, be conscious of gluttonous eating of animal foods and animal products. Research[20] has shown that eating animal foods and animal products and fats can have detrimental effects on human health if eaten in large quantities and too often and without ample vegetables.

Support your food's absorption with fermented products like sauerkraut, miso, umeboshi plums, and tamari, a gluten-free soy sauce—traditional foods from around the world that embrace health and healing. Although these might not be common where you live, all have good health properties.

Provide an appealing aesthetic at mealtime. Serve your food on pleasing plates and bowls, bring the family together, and promote a harmonious eating experience.

Learn to use a variety of cutting and cooking techniques, such as matchsticks or chunks, and pressure-cooking, light steaming, or sautéing.

Be aware of the five tastes: salty, sweet, bitter, pungent, and sour.

Prepare raw and sprouted foods and vegetable juices to provide the freshest naturally occurring vitamins.

Choose lunch as your main meal, because a light meal three hours before sleep provides a more restful night.

Finally, even with all this good food, it is still of utmost importance that you *chew each mouthful thoroughly*, as digestion begins in the mouth.

How to Make an Easy Transition

So, how are you going to get started on natural food awareness in your kitchen, and how are you going to make it an integral part of your daily habits? Here are some suggestions.

Keep a Food Journal—Gather Information!
The food journal is a powerful lifestyle tool to bring awareness of your eating patterns and habits, before you even start the journey of revamping them. Get a journal that you can carry around everywhere you go. Be honest, and don't judge yourself.
- Keep a record of what, when, and how much you eat and drink every day for one week. Be specific. Is it a complete meal with a variety of foods, or just a snack?
- How long does it take you to eat your meal? Do you drink as you eat? Do you chew and savor your food, or simply swallow it?
- Estimate the portions you are eating in cups or ounces. Do you take seconds?
- Write down how you feel after your meal and how you feel hours later, including both your emotional and physical feelings.
- Notice how you prepare your meals. How is your posture?
- How often per week do you eat out? What kinds of restaurants are you visiting? What do you order? Do you eat the bread they offer? Do you drink cold water during your meals?

Evaluation, Not Judgment!
After one week, you will have a pretty good idea about your eating habits. You might notice that you eat a lot of sugar-filled and refined foods, or that you eat meat and dairy at almost every meal, or that you all too often just grab a bite to eat without thinking. Are you hunching over the stove, stirring with tense shoulders, not breathing, and holding the phone as you cook by bending your head to your shoulder? Do you use a microwave oven, and if you do, how often? Do you eat in front of the TV or while doing other chores? What do you do after you finish your meal? Write down what you discovered about yourself. Don't judge, just start with Step 1 in this book and continue until you have mastered all 10 Steps. If you want, make journal entries during each Step and frequently refer to your early entries to monitor your progress.

How to Make This Transition with Your Family
If you have a family to cook for, don't make a big announcement like "We are eating healthy foods now!" The transition can be quite subtle. If you don't already do so, start by sitting down and eating at least one meal together without TV or other

disturbances. Increase the number of days each week when you create this precious family time where you share daily events and enjoy food together. This will make a big difference in the health of your family. Just cook the way you are used to, and slowly introduce new recipes, add more greens, and stop using sugar or refined and chemically processed foods.

Go to the farmers' market or nearby farms and harvesting times with your children or spouse and let them pick the vegetables and fruits they like. Have them help in the kitchen. Teaching children from an early age about where food comes from and how to cut vegetables or soak grains is important. Start growing some vegetables or herbs. Make simple food for small children, as they usually don't like mixtures of foods. It is challenging when you have teenagers, as they don't like to be different from their peers, but inviting their friends over for a healthy snack might be the way to begin.

Use your family's favorite vegetables more often, and don't force children and your spouse to eat everything you have prepared if they don't like some of it. You might have to cook two entrées sometimes, as all family members go through changes like this at different rates. Just keep on trying and do your best. And most of all enjoy yourself as you experience the bounty that becomes available to you and your family.

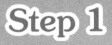

Step 1

Green Leafy Vegetables Are More Than Just Salads

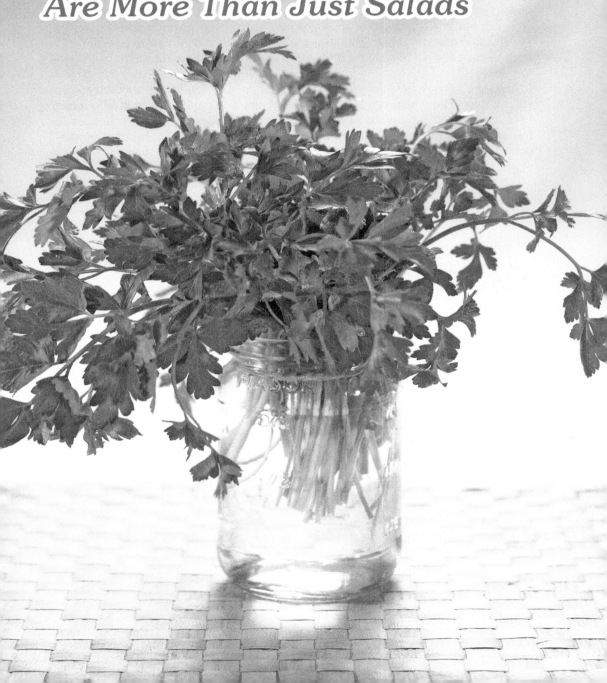

Your first step to a macrobiotic natural foods kitchen is to get into the habit of adding dark leafy green vegetables to your daily meals. Try to include at least one cup per day—and preferably three or more—during the first two weeks of creating your natural foods kitchen. This way you will become very familiar with preparing and eating these foods, and they will become a steady part of your lifestyle. Notice how good you feel after eating them for some time.

aWhen you ask people what they think is meant by "greens," the answers are typically spinach, iceberg lettuce, and other common salad ingredients such as green peppers. Many people are unfamiliar with the full range of green vegetables they can enjoy, especially the dark leafy ones that are very beneficial for our health. These greens are filled with nutrients and other phytochemicals—naturally occurring chemicals found in plants—that we need on a daily basis. They are easy to prepare, and they promote subtle, light, and flexible energy. Yet they are seldom found on menus or dinner tables. Men in particular eat very few greens—less than three cups per week.[21]

Start your transition to eating more leafy greens with kale. Just steam a few leaves for about three minutes and use them as a side dish or to top off a bowl of soup. When cooked, its flavor ranges from neutral to sweet. It has a very smooth, soft texture that is easy to chew. After trying kale, branch out to other kinds of greens.

Name Your Greens

If kale doesn't appeal to you, don't worry. You have many others to choose from. You can start with the ones you know, maybe broccoli, and then explore to find the greens you like best so you will keep on eating them often. Most kids and adults love to eat broccoli, so include it in your meal plans often. Use the stem as well as the florets, as you receive nutrients from both parts of the vegetable.

When you get bored with your favorites, be adventurous and try greens that you've never tasted before—or even heard of. Learn to recognize broccoli rabe, dandelion greens, bok choy, Napa cabbage, mustard greens, collards, watercress, or other greens from your vicinity, and add them to your meals. You can also mix your leafy greens with other green-colored vegetables like celery stalks, leeks, or green beans.

Complement your nourishing dishes with a variety of green herbs, if you enjoy their taste. These might be more familiar to you than green leafy vegetables, as herbs are most often used to enhance animal dishes. Use freshly minced parsley, scallions, chives, basil, mint, or cilantro as garnish or to mix in as you cook. Add fresh or dried thyme, sage, oregano, rosemary, or tarragon to bring the five natural tastes of sweet, sour, salty, and pungent to all of your dishes.

You can simply steam greens, snack on a few uncooked leaves, or prepare a raw salad from a wide variety of salad greens. Try nutrient-rich arugula, endive, chicory, romaine, wild greens, micro greens, or mâche salad (also known as field or lamb's lettuce). Toss cooked or raw greens with a homemade dressing of lemon juice, parsley, and olive oil, or prepare a pressed salad. More dressing ideas are in Step 8.

Seasonal Considerations for Eating Your Greens

Green leafy vegetables can be eaten every day throughout the year to provide nourishing energy for your body. Each growing season provides a wide variety. You can often find dandelion growing wild in your yard. If you are a gardener, plant seeds of your favorites and enjoy your own harvest, or go to a farmers' market for fresh produce. Natural food stores or your regular food store might provide locally grown, even organic fare.

Below is a list that provides you with a seasonal growing chart of most of the green vegetables found in a temperate climate. Depending on the climate zone you are in, these vegetables might be available at different seasons or have different names, and others might be available that are not on this list. All green vegetables can be included anytime into your meals, yet when they are in season locally, include them more frequently to support your health and your connection to the season and nature.

Spring	Summer	Late Summer	Fall	Winter
Asparagus	Broccoli	Bok choy	Cabbage	Brussels sprouts
Bibb/Boston lettuce	Chicory	Carrot tops	Celery	Cabbage
Broccoli	Chives	Chard	Mustard greens	Kale
Dandelion	Cucumber	Chinese cabbage	Scallions	Mâche salad
Green peas	Endive	Collards	Watercress	Watercress
Iceberg lettuce	Escarole	Daikon greens		
Parsley	Spinach	Lamb's quarters		
Radish greens	String beans	Leeks		
Ramps	Zucchini	Napa cabbage		
Romaine		Turnip greens		
Snap beans				
Spinach				
Spring onions				
String beans				

Nutrient Values of Green Leafy Vegetables

Pros:

- Greens are perhaps the most concentrated source of nutrition of any plant food. The health benefits of eating dark leafy greens are tremendous, including stronger immune and circulatory systems. Wild growing nettles and dandelion are helpful in minimizing seasonal allergies.
- Green leafy vegetables are loaded with minerals like calcium, magnesium, iron, potassium, phosphorous, and zinc; vitamins A, C, E, K; and many of the B vitamins. They are packed full of fiber, folic acid, and chlorophyll and provide a variety of phytonutrients, including beta-carotene, lutein, and zeaxanthin. Dark green leaves even contain small amounts of omega-3 fats.
- Lutein and zeaxanthin in greens will protect the eyes against cataracts and age-related macular degeneration. B vitamins, along with vitamin K, ensure a healthy nervous system, brain function, and healthy bones. Potassium and magnesium are linked to healthy blood pressure and blood sugar.
- Dark leafy green vegetables help purify the blood, improve kidney function, strengthen the respiratory system, and provide healthy intestinal flora. As green leafy vegetables are high in antioxidants, they might help to prevent some forms of cancer, as well as protect your eyes from age-related problems.

- Filling your plate with greens will help you eat less of the foods that could make you sick. Green leafy vegetables that are rich in calcium, such as kale or broccoli, do not contain oxalic acid, which could deplete calcium from your bones and teeth. In fact, the calcium in these foods is more readily absorbed than the calcium from milk and other dairy products. Instead of eating large amounts of dairy foods like milk and cheese that are not easily digested if you lack the enzymes to do so, or are lactose intolerant, eat green leafy vegetables to get your calcium.[22] A recent review[23] by Harvard nutrition experts stated, "a high intake of dairy can increase the risk of prostate cancer and possibly ovarian cancer." The Harvard experts also referred to the high levels of saturated fat in most dairy products and suggested that collards, bok choy, and baked beans are safer choices than dairy for obtaining calcium, as are high-quality supplements. The Harvard School of Public Health sent a strong message to the United States Department of Agriculture (USDA) and nutrition experts everywhere with the release of its "Healthy Eating Plate" food guide.[24] Harvard's nutrition experts declared that the university's food guide was based on sound nutrition research and, more importantly, not influenced by food industry lobbyists.

Cons:

- If you are dealing with certain health situations, caution is needed to make sure you are doing the right thing. Some greens, like spinach, Swiss chard, beet greens, okra, parsley, and leeks, are high in oxalic acid. These greens are eaten best with tofu, seeds, nuts, beans, or oils in order to balance the effect of the oxalic acid.
- The fibrous stems of greens are mostly not digested, but they provide bulk that is healthy for us. However, persons with very sensitive digestive systems, diverticulosis, or Crohn's disease should exercise caution when eating them.

Way of Green Life Inspirations

When you buy and eat organic and non-GMO foods, you keep harmful chemicals off your plate, and you protect future generations. Nonorganic foods may have pesticide or herbicide residues, and are grown using farming chemicals that pollute the water. Many chemicals can contribute to causing cancer.

Shop at your farmers' market to get your local greens, organic if possible, or start your own vegetable garden. You can easily grow your own kale, for example. It just needs full sun and a little compost added to the soil. Plant early (it tolerates a little spring frost) from seed, or purchase a six-pack of young plants at your favorite garden center. There are many kale varieties to choose from; consider, for example, dinosaur kale, a full, dark green plant. All varieties can easily fit into a flower garden or even in large decorative pots (not small hanging baskets, though). Amazingly, kale still grows after frost, and even gets sweeter! The leaves can be eaten cooked, made into chips (recipe in this Step), or blanched and tossed into the freezer for winter recipes.

There is no need to fear not being capable of creating your own macrobiotic kitchen with the right natural foods. Treat your body as a sacred place and feed your spirit with healthy foods and nourishing drinks. Keep your house in order and decorate it with large green leafy plants that provide good oxygen. Visualize a healthy new you, and step into your radiant, attractive, gifted, and wonderful self.

Things to Know When Cooking Your Greens

Look for fresh greens, and wash them as soon as you get them home by immersing them in water. Make sure to remove all the bugs. Finding bugs is a *good* thing, however, as it will tell you that these are most likely organic greens.

To store the greens, wash and then drain and dry them, wrap their stems with wet paper towels to keep them fresh longer, and put them into a chemical-free bag. If you have the space, put the stems into water, as it will extend their storage time. Slice the greens just before you use them, as they will lose their energy if their cells are injured and exposed to air too long.

Try a variety of methods like steaming, boiling, sautéing in oil, water sautéing, waterless cooking, or light pickling, as in a pressed salad. Boiling makes greens plump and relaxed. Bring water to a high boil and simmer them for less than a minute so they stay crunchy. Drink the cooking water, which should be a nice green color, as a health-giving broth or tea, or use it as your soup stock of the day. Steaming makes greens more fibrous and tight, which is great for people who are trying to lose weight. Leftover cooked greens should be stored in a glass or stainless steel container in a cool place. Avoid storing them in a plastic container (unless you line the container with parchment paper), as chemicals could leak into the food and thus change its energy and composition.

Raw salads or raw green vegetable drinks are also a wonderful way to enjoy greens, especially in the warmer seasons. These are refreshing and cooling preparations that supply live digestive enzymes. On a warm day, raw foods can cool you and thus help balance your energy. During very cold months, however, eating raw greens daily might weaken your energy, as your body could cool down too much. Small amounts of pressed or marinated salads that provide vitamins and enzymes for your digestive system can be enjoyed in all seasons. Green vegetables are also available in concentrated, dried powder form that dissolves in water. Stock up on these and drink a green drink when you are not able to prepare fresh greens.

Greens are powerhouses of nutrition. Eat them regularly to get fiber, vitamins, minerals, and many other nutrients that support well being. Add a dish of greens to each meal: steamed quickly in a covered pot, with or without a steamer tray, and a small amount of spring water.

Recipes for Green Leafy Vegetables

Quick Steamed Leafy Greens for All Seasons

Adjustable servings

Greens filled with chlorophyll will help your body greet the day with energy. Eating them is like taking in a burst of sunlight. Eat several servings each day. You can even have them for breakfast. Prepare what is in season like kale, collards, turnip greens, Swiss chard, spinach, mustard greens, daikon greens, broccoli, cabbage, Chinese (Napa) cabbage, or watercress.

Ingredients:
1 bunch green leafy vegetable
Filtered or spring water
Pinch sea salt
Dressing: drizzle of lemon juice and extra virgin olive oil

Preparation:
1. Wash greens: fill the sink with water and move them around, repeating the process until all the dirt is gone. Remove and drain.
2. Cut away harder stems from the leaves and slice separately, as they might need longer cooking than the leaves. Or use stems for soup stocks. If the stems are small, there is no need to remove them.
3. In a stainless steel pot, add water and just one pinch of sea salt. Insert a stainless steel steamer and bring the water to a boil.
4. Add the stems of the greens (if using) and steam them for two minutes. Add leaves and steam them for a few minutes with the cover on. The greens should be cooked but still bright and crispy.
5. Quickly transfer to a serving dish to prevent overcooking. In summer, dip the vegetables in cold water to preserve their green color.
6. Serve with your meal as is or seasoned with lemon juice and olive oil, or look under Step 8 for dressings.

Variations:
- Cooking option: Plunge a handful of greens at a time briefly into 1 cup of boiling water with a pinch of sea salt, and remove with a slotted spoon.
- Use a mix of 2 or 3 greens like kale, collards, and broccoli.
- Add slices of carrots for color and flavor, or invent your own creations.

Green Leafy Vegetable Rolls

Adjustable servings

These green rolls are great finger foods—no knives or forks needed! They can be served at parties, packed into lunchboxes, taken on trips, or just nibbled on as a snack. They are so refreshing. Children love to eat them and also like to help in the kitchen making them.

Ingredients:

½ head Chinese (Napa) cabbage or bok choy
1 bunch collard greens
3 carrots, washed
Several inches filtered or spring water
Pinch sea salt; Bamboo sushi mat for rolling
Seasoning per roll: ¼ teaspoon umeboshi paste (other options: mustard, sauerkraut, pickles)
Dip: mix tamari, wasabi paste (Japanese horseradish), and juice from grated ginger, to taste.

Preparation:

1. Wash collard greens and remove stems entirely. Separate the leaves from the Chinese cabbage and wash.
1. In a wide pot, bring 1 inch water to a boil with a pinch of sea salt.
1. Place several leaves of collards flat in the water and simmer for a few minutes. Remove the leaves carefully so they don't fall apart, and lay them out flat to cool. Continue until all are steamed. Slice carrots, steam, and set aside.
1. Repeat the same procedure with the Chinese cabbage, but boil for only 1–2 minutes.
1. On a bamboo sushi mat, place 3–4 leaves of collard greens. Overlap them and arrange them so they form a somewhat oblong shape. If you don't have a mat, arrange them on a cutting board.
1. Stack 3 or 4 Chinese cabbage leaves on top of the collard leaves.
1. Spread the umeboshi paste (or other seasoning) evenly in a line in the middle of the leaves. Layer carrots on top.
1. Start lifting the sushi mat and roll the vegetables into a cylinder, making sure that the collard leaves are tucked in and closing all around. (If you are rolling by hand, press and tuck the collards as you lift them so they stick together at the end and don't open up.)
1. Press the sushi mat with the greens inside to remove the remaining liquid. This helps the ends stick together.
1. Cut the roll into even pieces. Arrange them on a serving platter, and serve with the dip alongside.

Variations:

•   Place a variety of vegetables within the roll, such as cucumber, watercress, or scallions. Other good additions are pan-fried tofu or tempeh, or cooked beans and grains.

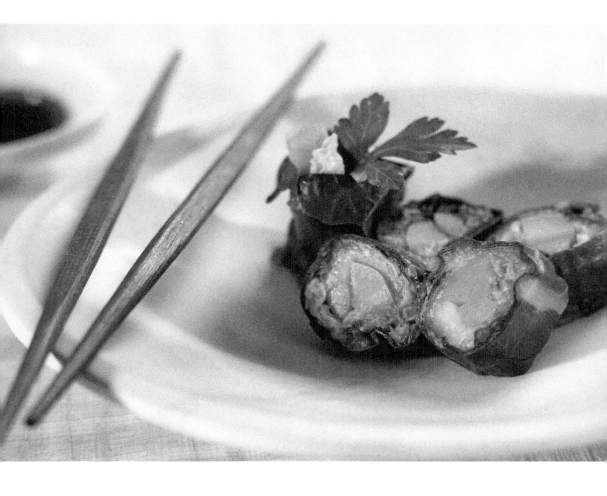

Nabe-style Vegetable Cooking

Adjustable servings

Nabe, pronounced "nah-bay," is a quick and light Japanese summer cooking style. Use a large open ceramic or stainless steel metal pot for this dish. Prepare it at your kitchen table on a portable burner and let people serve themselves, or cook it on the stovetop and transfer the pot quickly to the table.

Vegetable ingredients:

Choose a few leaves per person from a variety of greens like kale, Napa or Chinese cabbage, watercress, a handful of snap peas or snow peas, sprouts, and sliced scallions.

Broth ingredients:

3-inch piece kombu sea vegetable
3 dried shiitake mushrooms
½–1 cup filtered or spring water

Dipping sauce: mix to taste tamari, juice of grated ginger, minced scallions

Preparation:

1. Wash vegetables and slice into bite-size pieces. Group each kind on a platter and set aside.
2. Soak kombu and shiitake mushrooms for about 10 minutes in ½ cup water.
3. Remove and discard shiitake stems, and slice mushrooms and kombu into small pieces.
4. Pour ½ cup fresh water plus the kombu and mushroom soaking water into a large pot and bring to boil. Simmer for 10 minutes. This makes your broth. No other seasonings are needed.
5. Bring broth to a boil again and add each vegetable group in order according to hardness, so that each has its proper cooking time, usually no more than 1 or 2 minutes.
6. Toward the end add the sprouts or scallions, which require only several seconds of cooking.
7. Continue adding fresh vegetables to be cooked as needed, and add more water if needed, as the broth will cook away.
8. Serve vegetables immediately, while the color is still bright green.
9. Dip the vegetables into a small cup of dipping sauce before eating.
10. Variations:
11. Include finely sliced carrots or other root and round vegetables of your choice.
12. Add fresh tofu to the dish. Drink the leftover broth.

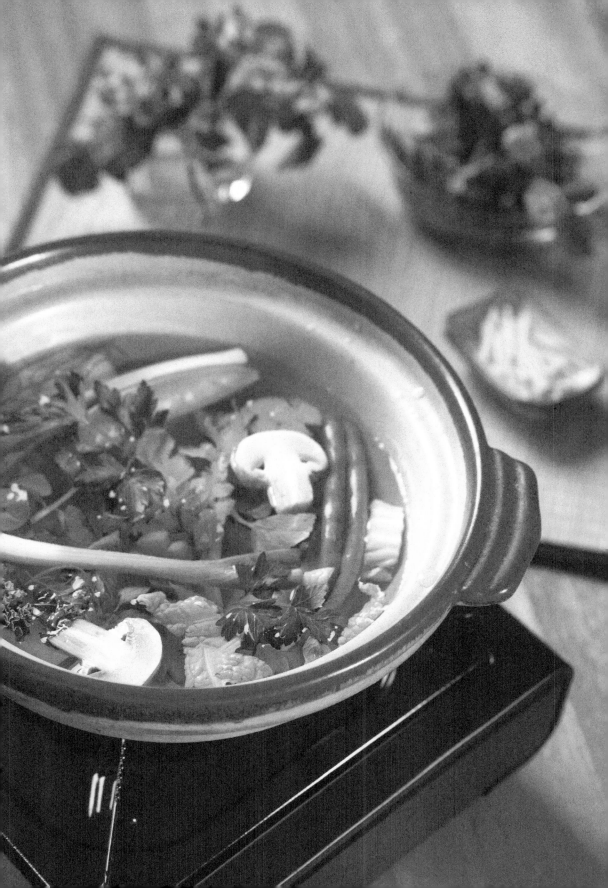

Kale with Golden Raisins and Toasted Almond Slivers

4 servings

Everybody, including kids, loves this combination. It is a great introduction to eating green leafy vegetables, as it blends sweet and nutty flavors. This makes a lovely dish for a festive occasion or a dinner party.

Ingredients:

3–5 cups kale
4½ cups filtered or spring water
Pinch sea salt
1 tsp. extra virgin olive oil or sesame oil
1/3 cup raisins
2 cloves garlic, minced (optional)
¼ cup toasted almonds, slivered
Pinch sea salt or to taste

Preparation:

1. Wash kale and roughly chop the leaves, or use desired cut.
2. Optional: if stalks are large, strip them from the leaves and slice and boil a few minutes longer.
3. Bring water to a boil and add a pinch of sea salt.
4. Dip the leaves into the boiling water and blanch them for about 3 minutes.
5. Remove, drain, and set aside. Save the cooking liquid to drink or use as soup stock.
6. Heat a skillet and add oil to coat. Add raisins and sauté 1–2 minutes until they puff up.
7. Add garlic, if using, and stir constantly to prevent garlic from burning. Remove from skillet.
8. Optional: toast almonds in the same pan until light brown.
9. Combine greens, raisins, and almonds in a bowl, mix, and add sea salt to taste if needed.

Variations:

• Use a few drops of water instead of oil to sauté the raisins.
• Instead of almonds, add walnuts or other nuts, or sunflower, pumpkin, or sesame seeds.
• Replace raisins with currants or your favorite seasonal dried fruit.
• Use other green vegetables like collards or broccoli.

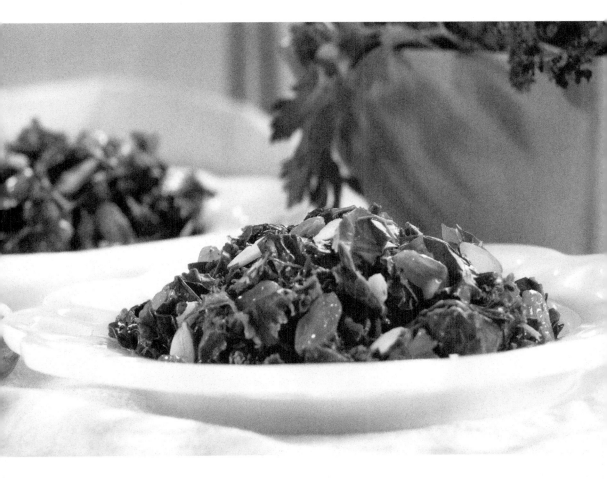

Dinosaur Kale Chips

4 servings

To forget how to dig the earth and to tend the soil
is to forget ourselves.
Mohandas K. Gandhi

Dinosaur kale is a beautiful, full, dark green plant that can easily fit into a flower garden or even large decorative pots. Amazingly, kale still grows after frost, and even gets sweeter! The leaves can be eaten cooked, made into chips, or blanched and tossed into the freezer for winter recipes.

Ingredients:
1 bunch dinosaur kale
Sprinkles of sea salt
Light drizzle of extra virgin olive oil

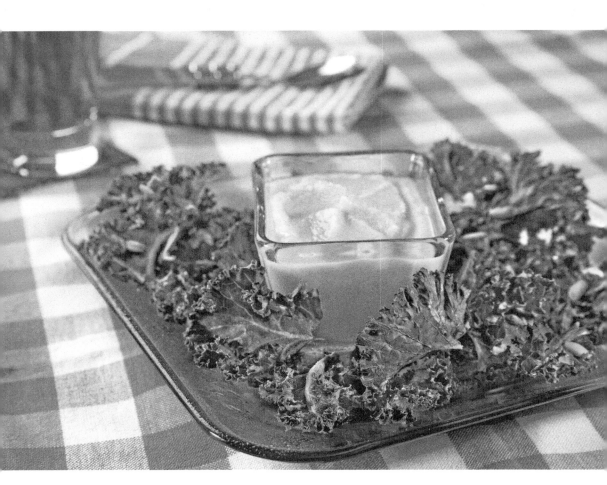

Preparation:
1. Preheat oven to 250° F.
2. Wash kale and remove stems.
3. Tear leaves into chip-size pieces.
4. Spin dry, or blot with a clean kitchen towel.
5. Toss in a large bowl with a very light drizzle of olive oil and sprinkle of sea salt.
6. Spread on a baking sheet or glass-baking dish in a single layer (small overlaps are fine).
7. Bake 20–30 minutes. Even if they look damp, they are probably done.
8. Use a fork or tongs to test. A little too much heat or extra time in the oven and the quality decreases fast.

Variations:
Serve with a side of roasted pumpkin, sesame, or sunflower seeds.

Instead of sea salt, add spices like garlic powder, chili powder, or smoked salt before baking.

Miso Greens with Daikon Radish

4 servings

This dish combines three dynamic nutritional foods. Miso with its great flavor is known for its enzymatic power. Daikon radish has strong detox qualities. Greens provide overall well being.

Vegetable ingredients:
¼ tsp. light sesame oil
1 cup scallions, finely sliced, with a few set aside for garnish
2 cups white daikon radish or red radishes
Few tbsp. filtered or spring water, or more if needed
2 cups kale or green daikon tops

Dressing ingredients:
1 cup finely grated carrots
1 tbsp. chickpea or light rice miso, mixed with 2 tbsp. warm water
1 tbsp. maple syrup
¼ tsp. grated ginger juice

Garnish: sliced scallions

Preparation:
1. In a small bowl, mix dressing ingredients together and set aside.
2. Scrub radish with a vegetable brush (don't peel if organic), and cut into small cubes.
3. Wash kale greens and chop into bite-size pieces, then towel or drip-dry.
4. Wash and slice scallions into small pieces, then towel or drip-dry.
5. Heat a large deep skillet or pan, distribute oil evenly, and turn heat to medium.
6. Sauté scallions for one minute then add the radish cubes and lightly brown.
7. Add 2 tbsp. of water and simmer until soft, 4 minutes or less, depending on the size of the cubes.

8. Add the dressing and mix, then place the greens on top and simmer for 5 minutes or less.
9. Add more water if needed. Mix and adjust seasoning to taste.
10. Serve garnished with fresh sliced scallions.

Variations:

- Sauté your vegetables with water instead of oil.
- Replace kale with your favorite green leafy vegetable.
- Add ¼ tsp. pressed garlic instead of ginger juice to prepare the dressing.

Sautéed Leafy Vegetable with Curry

4 servings

Tasty greens like kale, mustard, daikon greens, watercress, and bok choy are excellent sources of iron, calcium, and folic acid. Seasoned with spices and herbs from around the world, they provide interesting additions to your meals.

Ingredients:

1 bunch kale or collards
1 tbsp. sesame oil
1 cup onion, finely diced (optional)
¾ pound carrots, diced
Filtered or spring water, or coconut milk
2 cloves garlic, pressed or minced (optional)
2 tbsp. curry powder, or to taste
Pinch sea salt
1 tbsp. maple syrup

Garnish: chopped fresh cilantro

Preparation:

1. Wash greens.
2. Remove stems and set aside for a soup stock. Cut leaves into half-inch strips.
3. Heat the sesame oil in a skillet and sauté onion over medium-high heat until it starts to brown.
4. Add the carrots and half cover with water or coconut milk.
5. In a small bowl, mix garlic (if using), curry powder, sea salt, and maple syrup. Stir this into the pot and bring to a quick boil.
6. Reduce heat, cover, and simmer 5 minutes or until carrots are mostly soft.
7. Add greens and cook for another 3 minutes or until everything is tender.
8. Adjust seasoning. For a stronger taste, stir in more curry powder and simmer until most of liquid is absorbed.
9. Serve with freshly chopped cilantro.

Variations:

- Use a different seasoning mixture instead of curry.
- Try tamari and lemon, or spicy chili.

Refreshing breakfast drink, or anytime during the day

Blended Green Vegetable Drink

1–2 servings

Raw green vegetable drinks (juices or smoothies) provide quick and refreshing energy, and can bring relief from various conditions. Choose vegetable juices over fruit juices, as they won't spike your blood sugar as fruit juices might. Start juicing in the spring to eliminate heavy winter food, thus helping to prepare you for the summer season. For a liver detox, add dandelion and daikon radish. For a cold remedy, add ginger or garlic. See Steps 7 and 10 for more vegetable drinks. During hot summer days, vegetable juices can cool you down.

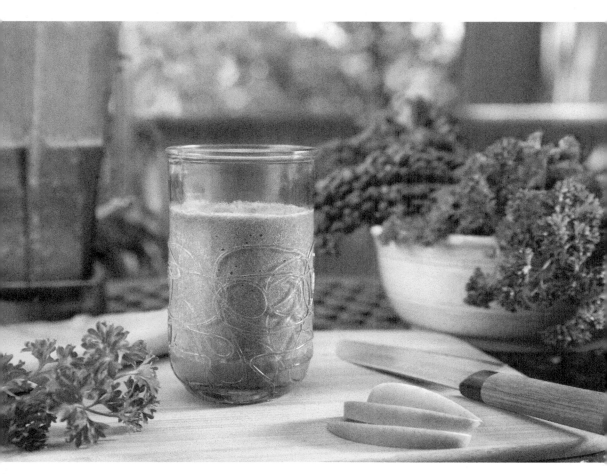

Ingredients:
6 kale leaves
2 collard leaves
½ cucumber
¼ cup parsley
4 celery stalks
1-2 green apples or other seasonal fruit
½ organic lemon, including the peel
1-inch piece ginger, or to taste (optional)
Filtered or spring water, or fruit juice, as needed

Preparation:
1. Wash all vegetables and cut them into pieces. There are three possible ways to make a green drink:
2. Juicing: Process everything through a vegetable juicer to get the nutrient-packed liquid. Drink fresh at room temperature, or warm lightly. Use the remaining pulp as a soup stock, or drink (see below), or compost.
3. Pulp stock: Place the pulp directly into a pot and add about one inch water above it. Heat the water and remove from heat just before it boils—about 180° F—to extract the rest of the nutrients. Pour into a strainer and push out as much of the liquid as possible by hand or with a pestle. Use as soup stock, or drink as is. Toss the remaining pulp into the compost bin.
4. Blending: Use a heavy-duty blender to achieve a thicker, smoothie-like texture with both juice and pulp. Add water or fruit juice to get the desired texture, if needed. Drink less, as the pulp will fill you up quicker.

Variations:
• Add whatever you have at home, or try carrots, beets, oranges, or other fruits and vegetables plus some liquid—water or fruit juice.

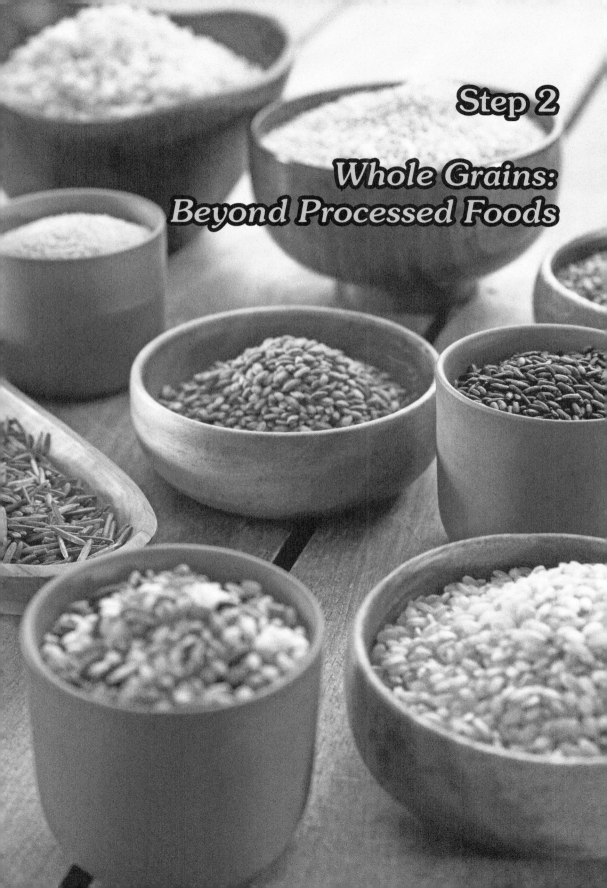

Step 2

Whole Grains:
Beyond Processed Foods

During Step 2, you will learn about the role that whole grains can play in your natural foods kitchen. Take the next two weeks to concentrate on studying the information and preparing the recipes. Continue using the green leafy vegetables recipes from Step 1.

Whole grains that have not been altered and are farmed sustainably and organically can be the best crops to feed the people of the world. The macrobiotic principle "one grain, ten thousand grains" tells how each single kernel of grain, when planted, can produce more seeds, and these seeds can also be planted to produce further seeds to be planted. Since one grain can produce ten thousand grains, having a good grain seed to start with is important. GMO-free whole grain seeds can be stored for many years, as they don't lose their power to reproduce. Grains found in ancient archeological sites, when planted, can still germinate.

Whole grains belong to the Poaceae family of plants, the true grasses. Eating these grains in their whole, unprocessed form can give you more stamina and energy. Their endosperm is our major source of complex carbohydrates, and many other important nutrients are found in the germ and seven bran layers. Whole grains are also called "brown," as in the case of brown rice, although the French term, riz complet, is a more apt description. They are complete whole foods, and when cooked, very healthy to eat.

In contrast, refined grains like white rice or white wheat flour (contains gluten) have had many of the seven layers of bran and the germ removed, and are thus also missing much of the fiber, protein, vitamins, and minerals that are present in those layers. Sometimes vitamins and minerals are added back into grain products, such as bread or breakfast cereal, which are then labeled "enriched," but these added nutrients are only a handful of the many phytochemicals that are lost in the refining process and don't make up for what has been removed. This substantial nutritional difference between whole grains and refined grains is important to note. Refined grains and white flour products are denatured and empty foods without much of the accompanying nutritional value present in the whole grain. Yet these empty white flour products are used in most commercial white breads and pastries, and are enhanced with white sugar and chemicals. Many ailments, such as diabetes, cancer, or heart disease, feed on such fare.

History of Whole Grain Eating around the World

Historically, hunter-gatherers have cultivated whole grains. Growing these crops ultimately led them to settle into farming communities. Some grains have been around for thousands of years, and cultures all over the world still enjoy them as primary foods. Barley was a staple of ancient Greece, Rome, Egypt under the pharaohs, and the Holy Land during biblical days, and traditional Tibetan society. In Europe, people traditionally used barley, rye, and wheat.

Recipes from the Middle East using wheat for pita bread, tabouli, and couscous have reached all regions of the world. Oats still have the status of a staple in Scotland, and corn has long been eaten in the Americas. Amaranth has been cultivated as a grain for about 8,000 years by the Aztecs. In India and throughout Asia, people traditionally used whole grain brown rice, but today, unfortunately, mostly white rice is eaten. In Africa, people still plant sorghum, millet, and teff, a grain native to the northern Ethiopian highlands.

Many peoples thrived on grain-like foods. Russians are known for buckwheat (kasha), and the Native North Americans for their wild rice. The Incas and other ancient civilizations of the Middle and South Americas used quinoa or canahua, recently rediscovered edible seeds.

Lost Traditions

Unfortunately, the more common and widely available corn and modern varieties of wheat and other grains have been bred over thousands of years to look and taste substantially different from their distant ancestors. They have lost some of their nutritional value and flavor. For instance, ancient barley, rye, and wheat contained much less gluten than is found in these grains today. We humans have not adjusted to these much higher volumes of gluten and have thus developed reactions that do not support the health of our species.

Fortunately, ancient, unadulterated grains with lower gluten content such as spelt, einkorn, emmer, and kamut have been rediscovered and are being grown commercially, and people once again have begun to embrace eating them.[25]

Name Your Whole Grains

Organic Gluten-Free Brown Rice and Its Many Forms

Mastering the production of a delicious pot of whole grain food will enhance your kitchen self-esteem. Try a bowl of brown rice. "Brown" rice, also called whole rice, with all the seven layers of the bran and the endosperm still intact, actually comes in many colors, sizes, and shapes, so you can easily prepare a number of amazing dishes. Brown rice does not contain gluten and can be eaten in all seasons. Experiment with short brown grain rice in the winter; medium grain brown rice, also called rose, in spring and autumn; and long grain brown rice, brown basmati, or brown jasmine rice during the summer. Branch out by adding whole black or red rice, and make dessert-like dishes with sweet brown rice. You can also mix whole red rice with short grain brown rice, for instance, or add other grains like millet, or beans like black beans, to introduce different nutrients, colors, tastes, textures, and energies to your table. To start getting used to eating whole grain brown rice, you could prepare a dish with half white and half brown rice.

More Gluten-Free Whole Grain Kernels from Which to Choose

Use amaranth, buckwheat, corn, millet, quinoa, sorghum, and teff, which can be added to your meal plan and provide exciting dishes for your family and guests.

Gluten-Containing Grains and Grain Products

Barley, bulgur, couscous, farina (cream of wheat), graham flour, matzo, semolina, seitan (wheat meat), triticale (a wheat/rye hybrid), wheat germ, whole-wheat berries, cracked wheat, white wheat flour, pearled barley, barley, rye, rye flakes, and bulgur all contain gluten. Beer made with any of these grains also contains gluten. All forms and varieties of ancient grains are wheat-like and contain some gluten: kamut, spelt, emmer (farro), and einkorn. Oats and oat flakes are generally gluten-free unless they are manufactured in a wheat-manufacturing facility. Be advised that many common household and cosmetic products also contain gluten.[26]

Eat Whole Grain Kernels on a Daily Basis

Let whole grains take center stage on your plate—it is said that humans developed their brainpower by eating them. Soaked and prepared properly and chewed thoroughly, cooked whole grain kernels provide the complex carbohydrates that will nourish your body all day long. Whole grain kernels also help to cleanse and balance your system. Home-cooked whole grain dishes can be eaten every day in all seasons. How much you should eat depends on your age, digestive system, and activity level. Whole grain kernels cooked from scratch are considered the most beneficial grains for your health. Master various whole grain preparation methods. Soaking the grains before cooking them yields the most nutritious and usable result, and neutralizes the phytic acid that inhibits the utilization of minerals. Start with simple boiling, and venture on to pressure-cooking. Pressure-cooking shortens the cooking time, preserves more nutrients, and makes the grain more digestible. Use the pressure-cooking method more in the colder months of the year, as it will provide you with stronger energy.

Eat Flour Products Less Often

If you wish to stay fit and healthy into old age, watch your flour consumption. When you grind whole cereal grain kernels into flour, they lose their nutrient content rapidly. Whole grain flour products also have a higher glycemic index than cereal grains in their whole form, thus influencing your insulin levels very quickly. Everyone should stay away from eating refined white flour products often, or omit completely. No flour products are recommended for diabetic people.

Besides whole grain bread, you can find a variety of products made with whole grain flour, such as pasta, breakfast cereals, cookies, crackers, muffins, corn meal or grits, whole grain tortillas or wraps, rice meal and flakes, and even grain extract drinks in natural food stores and markets. In your health-promoting natural foods kitchen, use such flour products, even if made with the best whole grain ingredients, only occasionally, say three times per week, or at social events. Within the range of flour products, noodles are the easiest to digest. Occasionally, to create a quick meal, use 100% buckwheat soba noodles, brown rice noodles, quinoa, or corn noodles.

Seldom eat whole grain flour products that are sweetened and contain oil, like baked pastries, muffins, cakes, and cookies, as well as crackers and chips. Use popcorn, puffed whole grains, and breakfast cereals moderately. The main reason to eat flour products only in moderation is that any flour product is absorbed quickly and thus raises blood sugar, and this insulin swing is responsible for inflammatory responses, increased tissue and cellular acidity, and a compromised immune system.

Gluten Advice: Wheat noodles, seitan (mostly wheat gluten), rye bread, wheat bread, couscous, rye flakes, and cracked wheat products like bulgur contain gluten. Many flour-containing desserts and snacks such as brownies, cookies, and breads can be found in gluten-free varieties, yet it's best to use these varieties only on occasion as well. These are also often loaded with sugar and fat to make up for the lost taste and texture that gluten provides.

Choose Whole Grain Breads over White Bread

Opt for unhulled, 100% whole grain, additive-free, and sourdough fermented and/or sprouted bread. Choose white bread for social occasions only.

A sandwich is quick to make and easy to carry around. Kids love a peanut butter and jelly sandwich for their school lunches, and it is also a favorite snack for many adults. In former times when bread was made with only good-quality whole wheat, it was eaten plain without butter, often with a bowl of soup, to provide energy and strength when farmers came in from the fields. The German grandfathers often made a soup for breakfast with hot grain and dry, stale brown bread crusts. These sourdough breads provide the benefits of the whole grain. Be sure to read the ingredient list and nutrition label and choose bread made with fewer ingredients. Sidestep yeasted whole grain breads, as most of the phytic acid remains in yeasted breads, preventing you from absorbing most of the minerals in the whole grain.[27]

Eating too much bread will make your mouth dry, so you could feel like drinking more liquid. We often suggest steaming a slice of whole grain sourdough bread in a vegetable steamer instead of toasting it, which makes it more digestible, and chewing each mouthful very well.

Gluten Advice: Most bread contains gluten when made with grains like wheat, barley, spelt, emmer, or rye. Choose gluten-free bread with the best ingredients if you have an adverse reaction to gluten, or omit completely.

Read the Ingredient Lists and Nutrition Labels
As with all packaged food, read the ingredient lists and nutrition labels to make sure that you are getting a wholesome product. Choose non-GMO (non-genetically modified) foods, and question the value of white, refined, and chemically enhanced breads and desserts laden with white sugar or high-fructose corn sweeteners.

Nutritional Values of Whole Grain Kernels

Pros:

- Whole grains, a central element of the human diet since the days of early civilization, are an excellent source of nutrition. Whole grains contain essential enzymes, iron, dietary fiber, protein, vitamin E, and the B-complex vitamins that are important for the hematologic and neurologic systems.
- Nutritionally, each grain is a bit different, just as individual fruit or vegetable species vary. They contain various amounts of the essential amino acids and other nutrients. You can alternate the grains, combine them with one another, or prepare them with a variety of beans and vegetables.
- Whole grains are most commonly known for their complex carbohydrate content, which provides you with more nutrition than refined grains or white flour products.
- Whole grains contain many phytonutrients in the germ and bran that provide important antioxidant activities and dietary fiber. Dietary fiber plays a key role in digestive and overall health.
- Because the body absorbs whole grains slowly, they provide sustained and high-quality energy. Eating them on a regular basis helps to stabilize the blood sugar and balance hormone fluctuations.

- Gluten-free buckwheat is high in minerals, especially zinc, copper, and manganese. It is heart-healthy, reduces blood cholesterol levels and blood pressure, enhances colon health, and discourages obesity. There are promising research findings about how buckwheat extract can substantially reduce blood glucose levels in diabetics. Buckwheat may be beneficial for managing diabetes.[28]
- Oats have many benefits: they can lower cholesterol and blood sugar and are an excellent food for persons with diabetes, rheumatoid arthritis, or hot flashes. For some people, however, eating cooked oatmeal daily can slow metabolism and increase phlegm, whereas whole oat kernels are better digested. Choose oats that are manufactured in a non-wheat-manufacturing facility if you are allergic to wheat, as cross-contamination can happen.
- If you eat gluten-free, choose the following grains: millet; long, medium, and short grain brown rice; brown basmati and brown jasmine rice; buckwheat; quinoa; wild rice; sweet rice, whole black rice and whole red rice, non-GMO corn; amaranth; sorghum; and teff.

Cons:

- Some grains contain gluten that may cause allergic reactions, especially when you often use milk and dairy foods. If you have allergies, are gluten intolerant, or have candida or celiac disease, you should avoid gluten-containing grains. A recent large study found that people with diagnosed, undiagnosed, and "latent" celiac disease or gluten sensitivity have a higher risk of death, mostly from heart disease and cancer.[29]
- Some individuals might experience reactions to other protein fractions like prolamin in grains, or other compounds that can cause similar undesirable effects on gut function.
- Studies[30] have shown that sugars and amino acids (asparagine) in certain foods form a compound known as acrylamide during high-temperature cooking such as frying, roasting, and baking. Acrylamide can cause cancer. If done for a longer period and higher temperature, larger amounts of acrylamide are formed, especially in French fries and potato chips, coffee, breakfast cereal, cookies, and toast.
- The main reason to eat flour products only in moderation is that any flour product is absorbed quickly and thus raises blood sugar, and this insulin swing is responsible for inflammatory responses, increased tissue and cellular acidity, and a compromised immune system.

Gluten Advice: Gluten-containing grains include wheat, barley, pearled barley, rye, and triticale, and their varieties—cracked wheat, wheat berries, bulgur, rye flakes, and the like. All forms and varieties of wheat-like ancient grains contain gluten, including kamut, spelt, emmer (farro), and einkorn. Some seasonings and condiments also contain gluten, like barley malt, barley miso, and soy sauce. Look at the ingredient list for gluten-containing seasonings. Rolled oats or oat flakes that are manufactured in a wheat manufacturing facility might be contaminated with gluten.

A Whole Grain Way of Life—Inspirations

*   You can get most varieties of whole grains in bulk bins or in premeasured quantities in bags at natural food stores.
*   Eating whole grains provides you with good nourishment and steady energy throughout the day. Brown rice provides the most centered energy, neutral taste, and sweet flavor, and is thus easiest to eat on a daily basis.
*   Cooking the right foods in your kitchen will help you and your loved ones to have enough energy to do good things. Involve your children from an early age in washing and soaking grains, thus teaching them healthy habits for life.
*   As health is more than just eating well, the daily way of life you choose can nourish or diminish you in the same way as the food you consume daily. Cultivate your sense of humor and create ways to live a happy life. Sing a happy song every day and give generously. Celebrate your success in the kitchen.

Seasonal Reflections on Whole Grains

Below is a seasonal chart showing you when eating each grain is energetically most beneficial to your health. However, you can eat any whole grain in any season, as grain has a central place in the vegetable kingdom and is one of the most balanced foods.

Spring	Summer	Late Summer	Autumn	Winter
Barley	Amaranth	Brown medium	Black rice, whole	Black rice, whole
Brown rice (boiled)	Brown basmati rice	grain rice	Brown medium	Brown short
Einkorn	Brown jasmine rice	Millet	grain rice	grain rice
Emmer (farro)	Brown long grain rice	Teff	Brown short	Buckwheat
Hato mugi	Corn, maize, popcorn		grain rice	Red rice, whole
Kamut	Quinoa		Red rice, whole	
Rye	Sorghum		Sweet brown rice	
Spelt				
Wheat				
Whole oats				

Gluten Advice: barley, pearled barley, rye, cracked wheat, wheat berries, bulgur, rye flakes, kamut, spelt, emmer (farro), and einkorn contain gluten.

How to Create Your Best Pot of Whole Grains

Cook Extra Grain

Plan ahead, as cooked whole grains keep well. Cook extra grain to use within two to three days of preparing it fresh. Cooked grains can be simply reheated in a vegetable steamer with some water, or prepare fried rice with good cooking oil, make rice balls, or add leftover grain to your soups. Serve grains with your favorite sauces, vegetables, and beans to create a complete, well-balanced meal. Use leftovers to make soft grain porridge for breakfast.

Soaking Grains Provides Real Benefits

In earlier macrobiotic literature you can find cooking methods that did not ask for grains to be soaked before cooking them. Not soaking produces an energetically more compact and stronger grain dish. Use this method when needed and when you don't have time to soak.

- Soaking makes grains more digestible.
- When you feel tense, try various methods of soaking the grain for a more relaxing dish.
- In a drier climate or season, soaking grains will provide more liquid to the body.
- Soaking decreases the phytic acid in grains, thus helping you to absorb more minerals, such as calcium, magnesium, iron, zinc, and copper.
- Soaking starts the sprouting process of the grain, which creates more phytonutrients, vitamins, proteins, and digestive enzymes.

- Soaking combined with fermenting for grains, flour, flakes, or meal, as in sourdough bread, makes the grain more digestible.

Several Methods for Soaking Grains

Different ways of soaking and cooking your grains provides variety in food preparation methods, another important aspect of healthy eating. Try several soaking approaches and compare with eating unsoaked grains. Find your favorite method, or use the one most suitable for the day. When you soak the grain, it will absorb some water and puff up, and thus less water will be available for cooking.

- Wash grain, and then soak in cool water up to for eight hours or overnight in a cool place such as the refrigerator. Replace soaking water with fresh water for cooking.
- Or wash grain, then soak and ferment with 1 tsp. acidic medium such as lemon juice or vinegar for each cup of water. Soak for about eight hours or overnight. Replace soaking water with fresh water for cooking.
- Or apply the cold water shocking method: bring washed grain to a boil and then add cold water to stop the boiling process. Repeat several times. Discard the water and restart cooking with fresh water.
- A shorter soaking time is OK when you don't have the maximum time to soak.

Water to Grain Ratio When Boiling Grains		
1 Cup Grain	**Water**	**Cooking Time**
Brown rice	2 cups	60 minutes
Buckwheat (kasha)	2 cups	20 minutes
Whole oats	3 cups	90 minutes
Rolled oats	3 cups	20 minutes
Quinoa	2 cups	20–30 minutes
Amaranth	2 cups	20 minutes
Millet	3–4 cups	20–30 minutes
Wild rice	2 cups	45 minutes

Note: If using a pressure cooker, time depends mostly on the type of cooker you have. Follow its instructions.

How to Cook Whole Grains

- Measure the grain, wash in cold water, then rinse, using a fine-mesh strainer. Choose a soaking method. After soaking, rinse the grain, put it in a stainless steel pot, and add the recommended amount of fresh water.
- As some of the soaking water is absorbed in the grain, your water measurement may need to be adjusted slightly downward, depending on your cooking method.
- Add a pinch of sea salt or a stamp-sized piece of kombu sea vegetable. However, do not add salt or kombu to kamut, amaranth, or spelt, since salt interferes with their cooking time.
- When boiling most grains, bring water and grains to a very slow boil, then reduce heat, cover, add seasoning, and simmer for the suggested amount of time. This way of cooking the grains provides a softer consistency. Occasionally check to see if more water is needed. When cooking buckwheat (kasha), quinoa, or amaranth, add the grain to already boiling water to create a separated, less mushy texture.
- After the grain is cooked, serve family style in a ceramic, glass, or wooden container, or put a couple of rice paddle-size or ice cream ball-size scoops onto each plate or bowl. Decorate with parsley or scallions, or sprinkle with gomasio, a sesame and sea salt mixture. See Step 8 for condiment ideas.
- The following recipes will introduce you to a variety of grain preparation methods, such as boiling, pressure-cooking (with and without a ceramic Ohsawa pot), soft cooking as for porridge, and light sautéing. You can easily interchange any of the whole grains in each recipe to create new variations. Experiment with using a rice cooker or slow cooker such as a Crock-Pot, or baking whole grain dishes in winter.

Recipes for Whole Grains

Boiled Whole Grain Brown Rice with Sesame Sea Salt Condiment

4 servings

Boiled whole grain brown rice makes a delicious addition to any meal, and it's a wonderful way to get acquainted with cooked whole grains. Plumper than short grain brown rice, medium grain brown rice is great to use in a paella or risotto instead of white rice. Boil it in a heavy stainless steel or enameled cast iron pot with a tight-fitting lid that promotes gentle and even cooking. Don't use aluminum pots or pans, since aluminum can give a metallic taste to the food and may have negative health effects.

Ingredients:
1 cup whole grain brown rice
2 cups filtered or spring water
Pinch sea salt
Garnish: Sesame/Sea Salt Condiment – Gomasio (Recipe in Step 8)

Preparation:
1. Wash the rice in cold water and soak for 8 hours.
2. Drain the water and replace with fresh water. (Or choose another soaking method from this Step.)
3. Place water, rice, and sea salt in a heavy pot and bring to boil on a high flame.
4. Reduce the flame to medium low, cover with a tight lid, and simmer for 50–60 minutes.
5. Check the water level periodically and add more if needed.
6. Remove to a serving dish.
7. Garnish each serving with sprinkles of Sesame Sea Salt Condiment.
8. Eat with a side of beans, greens, and a root or round vegetable dish.

Variations:
- Pressure-cook for approximately 45 minutes. (Pressure-cooking times and water amounts may vary depending on your cooker).
- Store leftover rice in a glass container with a proper lid in the fridge for 2 to 3 days.
- Use leftover grain in a variety of ways described in some of the recipes in this book.
- Instead of sea salt, cook with a stamp-size piece of kombu or half an umeboshi plum.
- For variety, add a handful of other grains like short grain brown rice, black rice, red rice, sweet rice, quinoa, or millet.

Fried Brown Rice Patties

4 servings

These fried patties are a wonderful example of the hundred and one dishes you can make with already cooked rice and other grains. They provide a great vegetarian alternative to a burger. They taste delicious on their own or in a sandwich—between whole grain sourdough bread, on top of romaine lettuce or a fried Portobello mushroom, etc.

Ingredients:

2 cups cooked short grain brown rice
2 tbsp. extra virgin olive or sesame oil
Seasonings: tamari, juice squeezed from grated ginger
Garnish: daikon radish, finely sliced raw onion rings
Parsley, minced

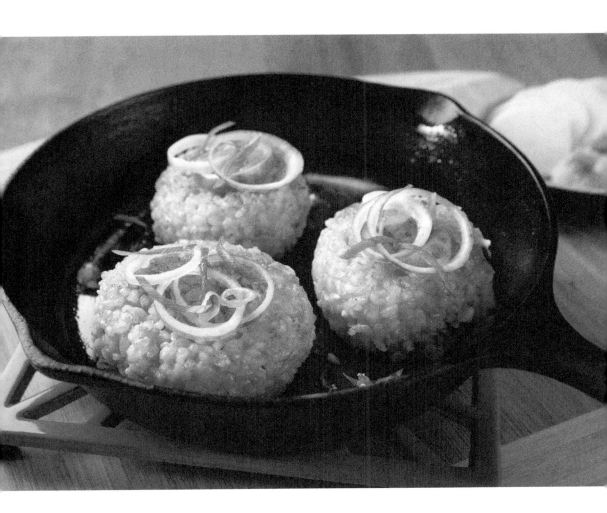

Preparation:

1. Form cooked rice into a firm patty with your hands.
2. Heat a skillet (cast iron works best), add oil, and place the patties in the hot oil. Fry on both sides for a few minutes.
3. Toward the end, when lightly browned, season with sprinkles of tamari and ginger juice.
4. Serve with slices of raw daikon radish or onions and parsley.

Variations:

* Add garlic juice instead of ginger juice toward the end of frying.
* Use the leftover grain mix from the Short Grain Rice with Sweet Brown Rice and Millet recipe.
* Mix in finely minced vegetables boiled for a few minutes before forming a patty. Add spicy seasoning or herbs of your choice.

Whole Grains Cooked in a Ceramic Pot

4 servings

Foods cooked in a ceramic crock always cook evenly without scorching, even if you cook just a handful. Best results are achieved if you insert the ceramic pot with a lid into a pressure cooker. For easy handling, use an Ohsawa pot, a Japanese earthenware pot named and designed by George Ohsawa, the founder of the twentieth-century macrobiotic movement.

Ingredients:

1 cup whole grain rice
¼ cup wild rice
¼ cup yellow corn
¼ cup green peas
2 cups filtered or spring water
Pinch sea salt per cup of grain

Preparation:

1. Wash grain and soak for 8 hours. Or choose another soaking method from this Step.
2. Drain the water and replace with fresh water. Place the rice, water, and sea salt into a ceramic crock or Ohsawa pot.
3. Place a plate on the crock or fasten the lid of the Ohsawa pot securely with the cord.
4. Place the pot inside a pressure cooker with about 2 inches of water in it to just half cover the pot.
5. Fasten the pressure cooker lid, place the cooker over a high flame, and bring it up to pressure.
6. When the pressure comes up, reduce the flame to low. Cook the rice for 45 minutes.
7. When done, turn off the heat and let the pressure come down naturally.
8. Remove the lid and take the ceramic pot out of the cooker. Open the cover and stir the rice. You can use the pot as a serving bowl.

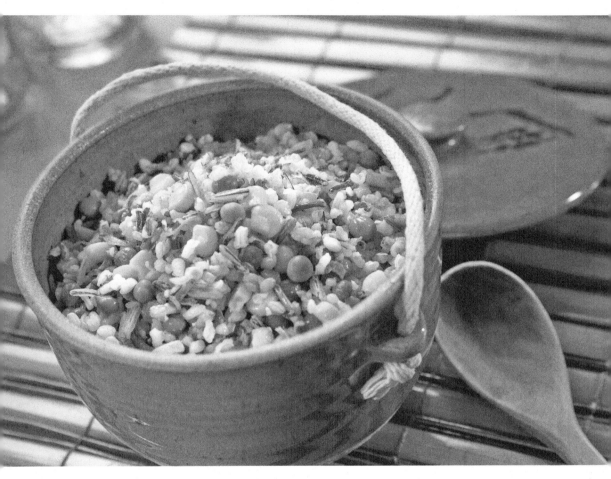

9. Leftover rice may be covered with the lid and stored overnight in a cool place such as the pantry or refrigerator.

Variations:

Use other grains, like 1 cup of millet and 3 cups of water.
Add a variety of beans to the mix, or use a grain mix.
Add vegetables, seeds, and nuts. Omit salt and add small piece kombu.

Pan-Roasted Millet with Teff and Sautéed Onions

4 entrée servings

Millet, with its golden-yellow color and tiny seed, is a delicious grain. It is best to roast it before cooking to deepen its flavor. Teff is a rich-tasting whole grain that comes in ivory or brown, with even tinier seeds. The homeland of both grains is Ethiopia. Teff flour can be mixed with water and fermented to make injera, a flatbread. These grains are both gluten-free and combine well with each other and with other grains.

Ingredients:
1 cup millet
½ cup onions, chopped finely
2 cloves garlic, chopped finely (optional)
2 tbsp. extra virgin olive oil or sesame oil
½ cup whole grain teff
Pinch sea salt
≈ 4½ cups filtered or spring water

Preparation:

1. Two options to roast the millet:
   - Wash millet, drip-dry, and then lightly roast.
   - Dry roast millet, rinse and then drip-dry.
2. Chop onions and garlic, if using, and sauté in oil.
3. Put millet, vegetables, teff, sea salt, and fresh water into a large pot. (Less water makes a drier millet dish, whereas more water makes it softer.) Mix gently.
4. Bring to a boil, cover, and then simmer 20–40 minutes, depending on the amount of water and the texture you like. When done, fluff the grain with a fork.
5. Serve with a side of fresh vegetables and a bean dish.
6. **Garnish** (optional): *Mushroom Onion Sauce w. Tamari and Ginger* (Step 8).

Variations:

- Leftovers can be formed into burgers and fried or made into pancakes with scallions.
- Soak the millet for 8 hours or overnight instead of roasting. Rinse and replace the water.
- Pressure-cook instead of boiling for a speedier preparation, 15–18 minutes.
- Add squash, cauliflower, carrots, mushrooms, seeds, or nuts to the grains and cook together.

Easy-going Buckwheat Noodles with Ginger and Scallions

4 servings

Protein, minerals, and antioxidants are all part of buckwheat's nutrient profile. When eating this popular buckwheat noodle dish, also called *soba*, you are not only stepping into the traditional Japanese cuisine, you are also building the list of your own family favorites.

Noodle ingredients:
1 package 100% buckwheat noodles
5 cups filtered or spring water
Seasoning ingredients:
Tamari, to taste
Juice from grated ginger, to taste
Scallion greens, finely sliced

Preparation:

1. Bring water to boil. Add the noodles, stir, and boil for about 10 minutes, occasionally adding cold water until noodles are slightly soft but not mushy.

2. Drain and (optional) rinse with hot water and serve hot.
3. In the summer, rinse with cold water and serve as a refreshing cold noodle dish.
4. Add tamari and ginger juice and scallions and toss.
5. Serve as a snack, appetizer, or hors d'oeuvre, followed with the main course of a whole grain, bean, and vegetable dish.

Variations:

*   *Soba Noodles in Kombu-Shiitake Dashi (broth):* Soak a 6-inch piece of kombu and several dried shiitake mushrooms for 10 minutes. Then bring to a boil in fresh water (or use the drained water from cooking the soba) and simmer 10 minutes. Remove kombu. Slice shiitake and add back to broth. Add vegetables or tofu and tamari/ginger seasoning to taste and simmer on low till soft. Serve broth poured over cooked noodles. Garnish with scallion slices, and add a sprinkle of wakame sea vegetable flakes (optional)
*   *Stir-fry Noodles:* Add cooked noodles to heated sesame oil and stir, adding garnishes like sliced scallions before serving.

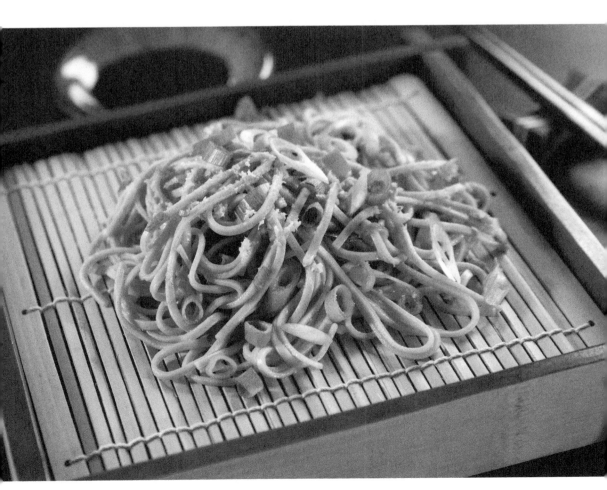

• *Gluten Advice:* Avoid buckwheat noodles that contain wheat flour, which contains gluten. Look for the noodle variety that contains only 100% buckwheat, as buckwheat is gluten free.

Savory Wild Rice and Vegetable Sauté – A Possible Holiday Stuffing

4–5 entrée servings

Wild rice is a traditional Native American food that is harvested in marshes in the northern part of the United States. It has a black to brownish color and a strong nutty flavor. Along with corn, squash, beans, berries, and maple syrup, it is a great introduction to American tribal cooking. Use as a savory stuffing for the Stuffed Pumpkin–A Possible Holiday Affair recipe from Step 4.

Ingredients:

½ cup wild rice
½ cup long grain brown rice (brown basmati rice)
2–3 cups filtered or spring water
Pinch sea salt
1 tbsp. extra virgin olive oil
½ cup onions, minced
2–3 cloves of garlic, minced (optional)
1½ cups carrots, minced or shredded
½ cake organic firm tofu, cut into small cubes (optional)
2 tbsp. tamari, or more to taste
2 tbsp. lemon juice, or more to taste
1½ cups snow peas, matchstick cut

Garnish: minced parsley

Preparation:

1. Combine rice and rinse with water. Soak for 4–8 hours, then drain.
2. Bring fresh water and rice to a boil, add a pinch of sea salt, cover, and simmer on a low flame 40–45 minutes. Fluff the cooked rice with a fork.
3. Meanwhile, wash and cut, then sauté in olive oil in the following order: onions, garlic (if using), carrots, and rinsed and towel-dried tofu cut into small cubes (if using), for about 10 minutes, or until carrots are soft; season with tamari and lemon juice. Add a small amount of water, if needed. Toward the end, add the snow peas and continue to sauté for another minute.
4. Remove from stove and toss the wild rice mix and vegetables together. Reseason if needed.
5. Garnish each serving with minced parsley.

Variations:

• Add organic corn to the mixture when in season, or other whole grains.
• Add a variety of other vegetables like celery or mushrooms.
• Cook this dish with beans instead of tofu.
• Add a variety of your favorite herbs and spices, or mirin, a sweet rice condiment.

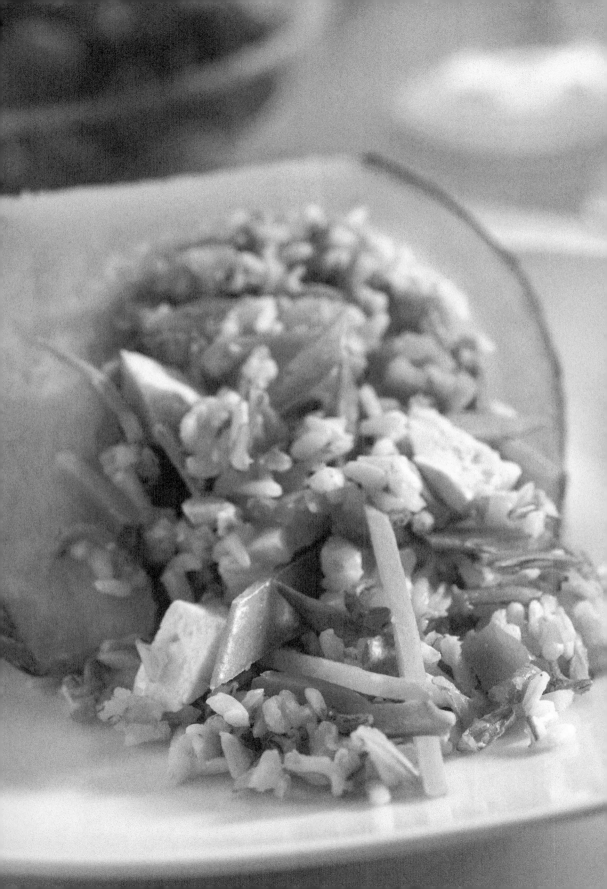

Quinoa Salad with Sautéed Vegetables

4 entrée servings

Quinoa cooks really quickly, is gluten free, and contains all essential amino acids. It is an ancient grain that has not been genetically altered. It is available in the colors yellow, red, black, and mixed, each providing a different flavor. Try them all, as they can bring a great variety into your cooking repertoire. Quinoa is great to eat during the warmer seasons.

Ingredients:

1 cup quinoa
2 cups filtered or spring water
Pinch sea salt
1–2 tbsp. extra virgin olive oil
¼ –½ cup red onions, minced
1 cup mushrooms, wiped with a damp cloth and cubed
2–3 cloves garlic, minced (optional)
½ cup red pepper, thinly sliced
1–2 tbsp. tamari or to taste
Black pepper to taste (optional)
1 cup broccoli florets, small pieces
Garnish: scallions, parsley, or cilantro, finely minced

Preparation:

1. Wash quinoa by rubbing it between your hands with water and rinsing thoroughly, then soak for 4 hours. Drain.
2. Heat fresh water. Lower flame, and gently add quinoa and a pinch of sea salt.
3. Bring to a boil and simmer uncovered for 20 minutes, or covered for a different texture.
4. Fluff the cooked quinoa with a fork and set aside, keeping it warm.
5. Gently heat the oil in a separate pan and sauté the onions and mushrooms till browned.
6. Add garlic, if using, and red pepper, and continue to sauté.
7. Season with tamari and if using, black pepper.
8. Add the broccoli and a little water, if needed, and steam for 3–4 minutes.
9. Remove from stove and toss the quinoa and vegetables together. Reseason to taste.
10. Plates or bowls of this dish look great when garnished with fresh green herbs.

Variations:

- Cook quinoa with teff, green peas, corn, edamame, or tofu cubes.
- Use your favorite fresh herbs or spices to create your own version of this dish.
- Season with a few drops of umeboshi plum vinegar to add a sour taste.
- Leftover quinoa tastes great at room temperature or heated the next day.

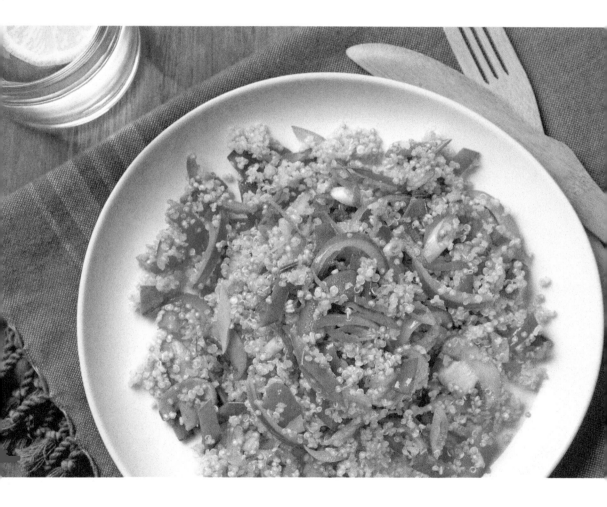

Healthy Breakfast or Anytime Dish

Soft Grain Porridge

2 servings

Research suggests that a healthy breakfast keeps you fueled throughout the day. It may also help your weight loss efforts. One of the most satisfying whole grain breakfasts is a soft-cooked millet or rice porridge, called *ganji* in Japan.

Ingredients:

1 cup cooked grain
2 cups filtered or spring water
Garnish: fresh blueberries, or other berries, or scallion/parsley mix

Preparation:

1. Use cooked grains from the day before like brown rice, millet, or teff, or cook fresh with ample amount of water. Optional: soak the leftover grain in water the night before.
2. In the morning, bring the water and grain to a boil, then lower flame and simmer for about 20 minutes. Toward the end of the cooking time, the grain should be creamy and porridge-like. Use a hand-held blender to make the texture even smoother.
3. Serve with garnish of your choice.

Variations:

*   *Salty-tasting porridge:* add ¼–½ teaspoon of miso paste diluted in a small amount of water, or for a sour-salty taste, add ¼–½ teaspoon umeboshi paste per cup of porridge toward the end of the cooking. Men like more salty porridge, whereas for women it should not taste too salty.
*   *Sweet-tasting porridge:* add raisins and nuts while cooking, and when cereal is soft toward the end of cooking, add a small amount of gluten-free brown rice syrup or maple syrup. Add (optional) unsweetened chocolate to taste. Children often like this taste. Top with fruit of your choice.
*   *Porridge with freshly ground flour:* roast ½ cup rice flour & teff flour mixed. Add 2 heaping tbsp. almond slivers, 2 heaping tbsp. raisins, a small pinch of sea salt, and about 1¼ cups of water. Bring to a boil and simmer for 10 minutes, stirring constantly.
*   *Healthy advice:* Only when in a real time crunch, use unsweetened boxed whole grain breakfast cereal with nondairy milk such as almond or rice milk.

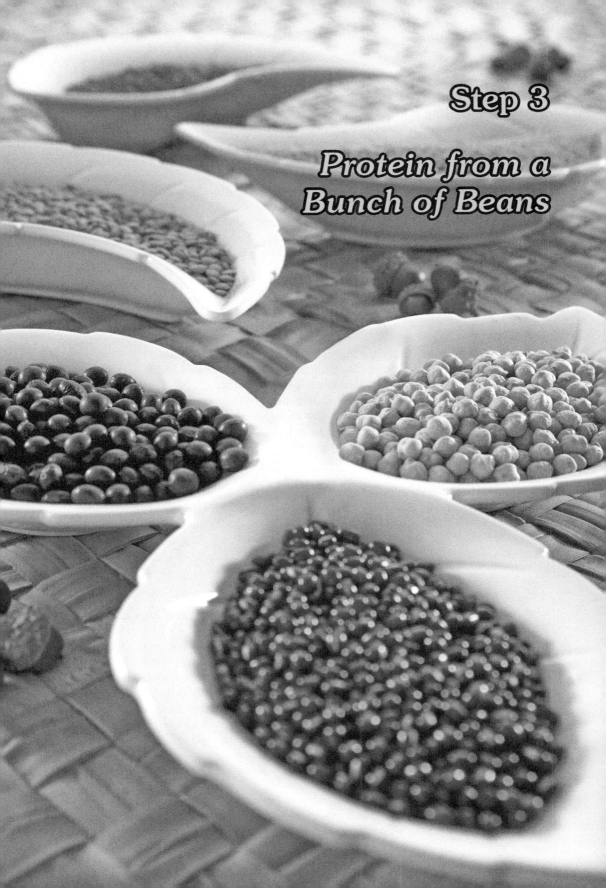

There are hundreds of beans for you to discover. As a wonderful way to
expand your cooking skills with high quality plant-based proteins, concentrate during
Step 3 on introducing a variety of legumes like beans, peas, and lentils as well as
seeds and nuts into your natural kitchen. Beans contain proteins that are building
blocks for healthy cells and tissues. Your body makes its own supply of amino acids,
but you also must get some from food. Protein comes in many different forms, and
animals and plants both contain it. What kind of protein you need and how much per
day depends on your age, gender, weight, physical activity, health condition, blood
type, and lifestyle.[31] Eating a variety of beans and legumes as well as unrefined
whole grains, seeds, nuts, and vegetables throughout the day will add good quality
plant-based protein to your diet.[32][33] A half-cup serving of whole beans or legumes is an
optimal complement to the other items on your menu. If you are not used to eating
beans, gradually increase the amount you consume. Most beans contain between
7–10 g proteins per half cup. A half-cup of split peas, for instance, contains 8 grams.

History of Beans

Archeological evidence indicates that lentils were already being eaten 9,500 to
13,000 years ago. Throughout history, many cultures cultivated beans and consumed
them together with cereal grains, because the hunt for animals was not always
successful, and therefore animal protein was rare. Native North Americans revered
the well-known "Three Sisters": beans, corn, and squash. In South America, early
cultures like the Maya, Inca, and Aztec used beans together with corn; by doing
so, they created protein dishes as nutritious as meat dishes. The Mexican cuisine
still uses beans with corn or rice. In India and other countries where the vegetarian
population is high, lentils and mung beans are among the many legumes that are
cultivated and eaten regularly. In most Asian countries, a combination of soy and
rice, and in the Middle East wheat products combined with fava beans, chickpeas, or
lentils, are used. In Africa, the indigenous black-eyed beans are a staple of the food
supply. Beans in Europe are small and come in brown or yellow shades; peas and
lentils are also commonly still eaten there.[34]

The Many Names of Beans and Legumes

Legumes are a class of vegetable foods found in great variety and cultural variation.
You can find them dried, canned, fresh, or frozen.

Fresh legumes like string beans, bush beans, sugar snaps, or snow peas don't need
long-time cooking and can be quickly added to a variety of dishes. These fresh beans
don't contain as much protein as dried beans; yet have other good nutrient content.
Favor fresh legumes that grow in season in your vicinity. Peanuts are also legumes
(not nuts); they contain a good amount of protein and are great to snack on or eat
occasionally as peanut butter with celery or on a whole grain sandwich.

Allergy Caution: peanuts can cause a reaction in some people.

As for dried beans, the same bean can have different names depending on the
region in which it grows. The small black bean is also called black turtle bean, black
Spanish bean, and Venezuelan bean. It is a common bean in South and Central
America, and is also popular in China, where it is fermented for many uses.

Then there are white and black soybeans, which are probably the most talked-
about beans. Asians and Westerners alike now use white soybeans to make products

like tofu and tempeh. The black soybean is a cousin of the white soybean—and higher in protein than the black turtle bean. Both black and white soybeans are considered vegetarian "meats" in Asia because of their complete amino acid profile.

Adzuki beans, also known as aduki beans or red oriental beans, are small red beans that are popular in Japanese cuisine and are often used to strengthen the kidney. Chickpeas, also known as garbanzos or ceci beans, are sold roasted and salted in markets and are the main ingredient in hummus and falafel, popular Middle Eastern dishes.

Another well-known category of bean is the lentil. Common types include light green, dark green (French lentils), red, and yellow, and all dals: mung dal, toor dal, masoor dal. These have been high-protein plant sources for centuries in India and Central Asia. The combination of brown rice with soybeans or lentils seems perfect for vegetarians concerned about protein intake. Both rice and legumes, bought in dry bulk, are very inexpensive and can be stored for long periods before cooking. Lentils are relatively quick and easy to prepare compared to other types of dried beans. All lentils, in whatever form, absorb a variety of wonderful flavors from other foods. You can use them in soups, salads, or baked goods and never tire of them. A serving of these protein-rich foods can replace a steak's worth of protein. Make lentils a staple in your plant-based macrobiotic and natural foods kitchen.

There are many other varieties of beans and legumes and peas to choose from—black-eyed peas, Great Northern beans, lima beans, navy beans, dried whole or split peas, kidney beans, mung beans, pinto beans, fava beans, Anasazi beans—and the list goes on.

Health Considerations and Nutrients in Beans

Pros:

- Whether vegan, vegetarian, or neither, everyone can benefit from adding beans to their diet. Eating a variety of beans and legumes daily will give you a high concentration of good quality plant-based protein. All beans and legumes are also high in iron, B vitamins, carbohydrates, and fiber, and are so versatile that you may never find them boring.
- Most beans are low in fat, calories, and sodium, high in complex carbohydrates and dietary fiber, and offer modest amounts of essential fatty acids. Only soybeans have significant amounts of omega-3 fatty acids, or oils in general. (For further information about oils, see Step 8.)
- Beans are extremely beneficial as an antidiabetes food because they rank low on the glycemic scale. This means that they do not cause the inflammatory, hunger-inducing spike in blood sugar levels associated with white potatoes, refined grains, simple sugars, high fruit juice intake, and baked goods.
- It is well known that the combining of beans and grains provides all essential amino acids. For instance, grains, which are lower in lysine (an essential amino acid), and beans, which are often lower in methionine (another essential amino acid), together provide a source of complete and high-quality protein.
- It was once believed that you needed to eat complementary proteins at the same time for your body to be able to use the amino acids. Then it was found that the

body is able to combine complementary proteins eaten the same day.[35][36] New research has shown that if you eat a variety of grains, beans, seeds, nuts, and vegetables on a regular basis on different days, you will still get all the essential protein.

Cons:

• Avoid giving most legumes to children under 18 months, because they have not developed the gastric enzymes to digest legumes properly. Small amounts of fresh peas and green beans are usually tolerated earlier.

Protein Content of Some Seeds and Nuts

Besides beans and legumes, all nuts and seeds provide your body with high-quality protein. Seeds like pumpkin and sunflower and nuts like almonds or hazelnuts contain a good amount of protein as well as nourishing oils, and they add satisfying tastes to many recipes. See Step 8 – *The Spice of Life: Seasoning, Oils, Sauces, Dressings, and Condiments* for recipe ideas.

• Almonds, ¼ cup ≈ 8 grams protein
• Hazelnuts, 1 cup ≈ 17 grams protein
• Peanuts, ¼ cup ≈ 9 grams protein
• Cashews, ¼ cup ≈ 5 grams protein
• Pecans, ¼ cup ≈ 2.5 grams protein
• Sunflower seeds, ¼ cup ≈ 6 grams protein
• Pumpkin seeds, ¼ cup ≈ 8 grams protein
• Flax seeds, ¼ cup ≈ 8 grams protein

Why Meatless Fare Is Becoming So Popular

There are several reasons why animal protein foods are being replaced more and more with vegetable protein-rich foods. One is that the farming practices for animals don't satisfy educated consumers anymore. All over the world, recalls and scares concerning this or that animal food are heard increasingly heard on the news, and health awareness is rising. Also, people are becoming more compassionate toward animals, and eating them is ethically offensive to many.

Another reason is research findings like those published in The China Study.[37] This book talks about some startling implications of food choices for diet, weight loss, and long-term health. It suggests that including more green and yellow foods and more vegetables in general, and eating less meat, can reduce the risk of diabetes, heart disease, and obesity.

Research has also shown that people who eat the most animal-based foods get the most chronic disease, whereas people who eat the most plant-based foods are the healthiest and tend to avoid chronic disease. These nutritional studies [38][39][40][41] also assure us that one can get a reasonable amount of protein by eating from only the vegetable kingdom.

High-protein meat diets are said to promote weight loss, prevent disease, and enhance athletic performance, but little supporting research exists. Studies actually suggest otherwise: a diet high in protein can contribute to disease and various health problems. A natural foods plate filled with a variety of whole foods—greens, root and round vegetables, sea vegetables, fermented foods, seeds, nuts, beans, complex carbohydrates, and healthy amounts of vegetable and/or animal proteins and fats—has been shown to be the healthiest on the planet.

Your Plant-Centered Kitchen and Animal Foods

Traditionally, meat was eaten rarely and often fermented to make it more digestible. In your natural kitchen, first and foremost fill your plates and bowls with a kaleidoscope of items from the vegetable kingdom.

The use of animal foods and products is up to the individual. If you choose to eat animal foods, use only small sensible amounts (health permitting), or enjoy on social occasions. Our most important suggestion is to select only wild ocean/ecosystem-friendly fish that are free of contaminants. As fish digests very quickly, more like vegetables compared to other animal foods, our recommendation for your first choice is small amounts of white fish like cod or halibut, and secondly, red meat fish like salmon. Fish is also the furthest food from humans on the animal evolutionary scale, making it a better choice if you are eating for spiritual development.

As for animal foods like red meats, poultry, eggs, butter, and all foods containing dairy, make a deliberate decision to eat only animal products that are organic, grass-fed, and humanely raised without hormones. Wild game is also a good choice. Eat these wisely in palm-size small amounts ($\approx$ 4 oz.), and when needed. To help digestion, serve them with a side dish of grated daikon radish or ginger with a drop of tamari soy sauce.

Three Methods to Consciously Choose a Meatless Lifestyle

If you are still eating animal products heavily and are interested in reducing or eliminating your consumption, here are several ways to do it:

1. Just include more vegetables, grains, lentils, and beans into your meals. You will thus naturally diminish your need for meat and reduce or remove the foods that are not as health supportive. Legumes can be a healthy substitute for meat, as they are low in fat, are a good source of protein, and contain no cholesterol.
1. Ease your way into a more vegetable-based lifestyle with a *Meatless Monday, Meatless May,* or *Meatless March,* or just be *meatless mindful* by reducing the amount of animal foods in general. Find people and groups that support your decisions.
1. If you really want to experience a difference in how you feel, you can take the *Meat-Free Challenge.* For the next two weeks, don't eat any animal foods, but continue eating well-rounded meals containing grains, beans, and a variety of vegetables and fermented foods, and carefully observe how you feel. If you like your results, continue eating seasonal, well-balanced vegetable meals. Remember, it is rare in this day and age in Western countries to be protein deficient.

A Few Words about Soybeans!
What Is Healthy—And What Is Not!

We know that soybeans have nearly twice as much protein as meat or fish, and eleven times as much protein as milk. Soy provides adequate amounts of all eight essential amino acids (protein content is 34%), which makes soy a complete source of protein. Soybeans also contain vitamins, minerals like calcium, phosphorus, and iron; lecithin; fat (18%), and carbohydrates (31%).

In Asia, the soybean is used mostly as a fermented seasoning or fermented soybean product. Miso paste, tamari, soy sauce (gluten-containing), and products like natto, tempeh, and tofu are used frequently in the traditional cuisines, but usually in relatively small amounts. Some research suggests that soy in these forms, along with green tea and other healthy lifestyle choices, plays a role in the lower incidence of breast cancer in Asian countries.[42] We also know that eating soy foods from early childhood on can provide protective factors later in life. Therefore, for the macrobiotic kitchen we suggest using soy in the same way it is used in traditional Japanese cuisine.

Healthy: Organic Non-GMO Fermented and Whole Soybeans

- Add small amounts of fermented miso paste to soups that also include sea vegetables and shiitake mushrooms and other vegetables, grains, or beans. Soybean miso (hatcho miso) has a very strong flavor, and therefore we often use a combination miso—soy/rice or soy/barley (contains gluten).
- Enjoy the flavor of fermented tamari or soy sauce (contains gluten) and season your dishes with a few dashes.
- About three times per week, include a small amount (¼ cup) of a fermented tempeh or natto dish. (One cup of tempeh contains 41 g protein.) Men should opt for these more yang soy protein sources and a variety of other beans instead of tofu, at least on a regular basis.
- Tofu is an easy-to-digest protein, because the tofu-making process removes the hull, where most of the bean's phytic acid is found. You will digest it even better when you eat it seasoned with fermented foods like miso or tamari. Use tofu (½ cup) about three times per week in miso soup, or as a homemade miso-fermented tofu cheese. (One-half cup tofu contains 20 g protein.) Use it only very rarely as a sweet treat or a sweet dessert for guests. For women, as you go through menopause, adding ¼ cup of tofu per day to meals may diminish the occurrence of hot flashes.[43 44]
- Edamame (fresh green soybeans) can occasionally be prepared boiled as a snack or cooked with grains.
- Roasted and salted soy nuts or roasted soybeans may be eaten as snacks.
- Enjoy properly soaked and cooked dried black soybeans or white soybeans as an alternative to other types of beans. Adding sea vegetables while cooking beans adds to the increased absorption of their minerals and their digestibility. Season with tamari or miso.
- In the process of "weaning" yourself from dairy milk, use unsweetened soy, almond, hemp, or rice milk in recipes or as beverages.
- Gluten and Allergy Advice: Barley miso and soy sauce contain gluten. Miso is also available without soy or gluten, such as in chickpea or adzuki bean miso.

Not Healthy: Processed and Refined Soy Foods

The recent trend in Western countries of consuming huge amounts of processed and refined soy foods as a high-protein alternative in plant-based diets has raised concerns. We have no long-range history of human consumption of these heavily processed (with hexane, a neurotoxin) isolated soy protein foods to look at. But some studies, as well as anecdotal stories, say these manufactured goods are not healthy.

- Avoid soy cheese, soy sausages and burgers, tofu turkey, soy "meat," soy chips, soy ice cream, soy yoghurt, and soy-based beverages. These are processed, refined soy food products that should not have a place in your natural foods kitchen. They might look or taste like the meat and dairy foods you used to eat or want to avoid, yet switching to them will be a huge roadblock on your way to a healthy lifestyle. These refined soy foods are only an artificial answer and mislead you into thinking you are eating a new vegetarian or vegan "healthy" product. Use all the Steps in this book to create a well-balanced plant-based lifestyle for yourself and your loved ones instead of relying on these processed soy foods. If you have an allergic reaction to soy, we recommend omitting all soy foods.
- If you want to experience plant-based food that tastes similar to meat, and are not allergic or have no adverse reactions to gluten, try protein-rich seitan that is made from wheat gluten. Seitan, also called "wheat meat," "mock duck," or "vegie beef," has a very high protein content and is a traditional food with a long history.

  Gluten Advice: Seitan and wheat meat have very high gluten content and are not suitable for people with gluten sensitivities or allergies. If you order vegetarian dishes in Asian restaurants with ingredients such as mock duck or vegie beef, be aware that those products are usually made from wheat gluten.

The Seasons of Beans

It is good to eat seasonal foods as you're balancing your meals with a wide range of produce, ensuring that you and your loved ones do not get bored. Eating certain beans throughout the year is a great way to strengthen some organs. For instance, adzuki beans are helpful to eat when you have kidney and bladder problems. Include them as a strengthening, healthy dish in any season. Do note, however, that knowledge of seasonal energies is helpful in choosing beans, just as with vegetables and grains. Eating winter food in the summer and vice versa on a regular basis is not advisable, as it will bring you out of balance. Below is a chart of beans in relation to the season in which each one energetically nourishes you best.

Spring	Summer	Autumn	Winter
Bush beans Dal, all kinds Edamame (green soybeans) Fava beans String beans Tofu Yellow & red lentils	Chickpeas Tempeh Yellow soybeans	Black-eyed peas Navy beans	Adzuki beans Black (turtle) beans Black soybeans Kidney beans

An Easy Way to Cook Dried Beans

- Measure beans, check for rocks and broken beans, then rinse. Soak for 8 hours or overnight, using 2–3 cups of water per cup of beans. Small and medium-size beans may require less soaking (4 hours). Older and drier beans often need longer soaking and cooking methods to soften them. See below for further soaking instructions.
- Drain the beans and discard the soaking water. Discard any loose skins before cooking, as this will increase digestibility.
- Place the beans in a heavy pot and add 3–4 cups fresh water. If using a pressure cooker, add 2–3 cups fresh water per cup of beans.
- Do not add salt at the beginning of cooking, only when the beans are about 80% done. If salt is added at the beginning, the beans will not cook completely.
- Add a small piece of kombu sea vegetable or a few bay leaves for flavor and better digestibility.
- Bring to a full boil and skim off the foam. Replace the removed water.
- Cover, lower the temperature, and simmer for the suggested time. Check beans periodically and add water if needed. Beans are done when the middle is soft and easy to squeeze. Larger beans such as garbanzos will usually need more cooking time, while smaller ones such as lentils will need less.
- When you use a pressure cooker, you can experiment with the length of cooking time and amount of water needed to cook different types of beans. Refer to your pressure cooker guidebook for advice.
- About 10 minutes before the end of cooking time, for either pressure cooking (after the pressure has come down) or boiling, add ¼ tsp. of unrefined sea salt per cup of beans and continue simmering. Salt is a digestive aid when used correctly.
- Finish your dish by adding combinations of ingredients and seasonings. For flavor variety, you can add rice miso or tamari near the end of cooking.

Things to Know about Beans

- Store dried beans in glass containers in a cool, dark place and use them within a year.
- To make beans more digestible, add a teaspoon of vinegar—apple cider, brown rice, or umeboshi—to the water in the last stages of cooking. This softens the beans and breaks down the protein chains and indigestible compounds.
- Adding fennel, cumin, savory, or bay leaf near the end of cooking, along with kombu as described above, helps prevent flatulence (gas).
- Experiment with your ability to digest beans. Smaller beans like adzuki, lentils, mung beans, and peas digest most easily. Pinto, kidney, navy, black-eyed peas, garbanzos, lima, black beans, and yellow and black soybeans are harder to digest and should be eaten only occasionally. Chew all beans thoroughly, and know that even small amounts have high nutritional and healing value.
- You can sprout your beans for even more digestibility and protein. Eat sprouted beans raw in a salad or cooked in a variety of ways.
- Pan-roast chickpeas or black soybeans instead of soaking.
- For convenience, use a can of precooked beans in recipes.

Several Methods of Soaking Dried Beans

Easy cooking tip: soak your beans at the same time you soak your grains. Cook them at the same time in separate pots, or combine in one pot for a delicious grain/ bean dish.

Soaking beans has some real advantages. A shorter cooking time is probably the biggest one, but soaking also leaches out some of the gas-producing properties and increases phytonutrients, vitamins, and availability of proteins. During soaking, beans will absorb water until they have increased in volume and weight about three times. Rinse your beans after soaking and cook them with an ample amount of fresh water.

- Soak in hot water for 8 hours or overnight, and add 1–3 tsp. of plum vinegar. This method will remove most of the phytic acid.
- Or just soak in water for 8 hours or overnight. Kombu may be added.
- Shorter soaking time is OK for some beans like lentils.
- If you forgot to presoak the beans but still want to use them in your meal, bring them to a boil in water to cover. Turn off the heat, add umeboshi plum vinegar, cover the pot, and let stand for one hour. Replace water and start regular cooking method.
- If you are really pressed for time, use a can of organic beans, or use the cold water shocking method. Wash beans, add water to cover, bring to a boil, and then add umeboshi plum vinegar. Add cold water to stop the boiling process, and scoop up and discard all the foam. Repeat this step several times before the final cooking, discard water, rinse beans, and add fresh water and kombu.

These cooking times are for boiling beans after soaking.

Pressure-cooking times will vary.

1 Cup Dry Beans	Boiling Minutes
Adzuki	60–90
Black (turtle) beans	60–90
Black-eyed peas	30–45
Chickpeas (garbanzos)	60–90
Great Northern	60–90
Lentils: brown & French	30–45
Lentils: red, yellow	20–30
Mung	60
Navy	60–90
Pinto	60–90
Split peas	45

Make Different Dishes from One Pot of Cooked Beans

- Cook extra beans. Cooked beans keep well for about 4–5 days, so you can cook extra and prepare a variety of dishes from one pot of beans. Freeze leftovers for use when you're crunched for time.
- Make patties. Drain excess liquid from beans, or add a small amount of flour to achieve a dry consistency. Take a handful of beans and press together. Heat sesame oil or other high-quality vegetable oil in a pan and fry each side till brown.
- Make a bean dip. At the end of cooking time, puree or mash the beans, mix in finely grated walnuts, and serve as a dip for slightly steamed slices of vegetables like carrots, celery, cauliflower, or broccoli.
- Try bean combination dishes. These are very savory, easily digestible, and wholesome combinations. Use your favorite beans to provide a variety of tasty experiences.
  - Use 20% carrots and onions to 80% beans
  - Use 30–50% acorn, butternut, or buttercup squash to 50–70% beans
  - Use 10–30% chestnuts to 70–90% adzuki beans or black soybeans.
  - Use 10% grains to 90% beans
- Prepare soups and stews. After your beans are cooked, add more water and boil them with chopped onions, carrots, and celery. Make a stew by adding kuzu to thicken. Add different flavors with your favorite herbs and spices.

Recipes for
Protein from a Bunch of Beans

Versatile and Multicolored Lentils

4 servings

Make this dish in the summer with yellow and red lentils that have shorter cooking times, about 15 minutes. During colder seasons, use brown, green, or French lentils with longer cooking times more often. In many of the bean recipes we use kombu sea vegetables to help soften the beans and make them more digestible. Lentil soups are easily prepared simply by adding more water and vegetables.

Ingredients:
1 cup green lentils
3 cups filtered or spring water
1-inch piece kombu, soaked 10 minutes
¼ cup celery, diced
½ cup carrots, diced (2 small)
3 cloves garlic, minced (optional)
1 tbsp. extra virgin olive oil
¼ tsp. sea salt
Dash umeboshi vinegar or apple cider vinegar
Garnish: sliced scallions

Preparation:
1. Wash lentils and cover with about 2 inches of water; soak 4 hours or overnight.
2. Drain and replace water, or use other soaking method from this Step.
3. Add 3 cups of water per cup of lentils. Bring lentils, water, and kombu to a boil and simmer for 30 minutes. Remove the cooked kombu.
4. Sauté the celery, carrots, and (if using) garlic, a few minutes in oil. The vegetables should still be crunchy. Add them to the lentils.
5. Season with sea salt and add seasonings of your choice (see Variations for ideas).
6. Optional: Add finely sliced green leafy vegetables at the end and let flavors blend for a few minutes.
7. Add a dash of umeboshi vinegar. Stir and simmer for 5 minutes.
8. Garnish with scallions and serve with a grain and green leafy vegetable dish.

Variations:
- Use seasonings like curry, turmeric, or cumin for an East Indian taste.
- Add European herbs like bay leaf or ¼ tsp. marjoram.
- Add tamari, or 2 tbsp. brown rice miso pureed with warm water for an Asian flavor.
- Add mushrooms or other seasonal vegetables.
- Mix with barley (contains gluten) or cooked quinoa for a hearty salad.

Three Bean Salad

4-5 servings

String beans, also called green beans or French string beans, are high in antioxidants like lutein, beta-carotene, violaxanthin, and neoxanthin. Use fresh green string beans freely in many recipes and add them to soups, or stir-fry them with other vegetables. Adding garbanzo and kidney beans to the string beans raises the level of protein in this dish.

Ingredients:
½ pound fresh green beans
1½ cup cooked kidney beans
1½ cups cooked garbanzo beans
1 tbsp. extra-virgin olive oil
¼ cup red onion, chopped
1 clove garlic, minced (optional)

Dressing:
2½ tbsp. red wine vinegar (or apple cider vinegar, umeboshi vinegar, or lemon juice)
2 tbsp. tamari soy sauce
¼ cup extra-virgin olive oil
1/8 cup Italian parsley or cilantro, chopped
Sea salt and freshly ground black pepper, to taste

Preparation:
1. Remove stems from green beans; pull off the strings, and rinse. Lightly steam until tender crisp, about 4-5 minutes, depending on size. Rinse under cold running water to stop the cooking. Cut into thirds and place in a medium bowl.
2. Add cooked kidney and garbanzo beans.
3. Heat pan, add one tablespoon of olive oil, and lightly sauté onions and garlic, if using.
4. Whisk vinegar and tamari in a small bowl. Slowly drizzle in the olive oil, whisking constantly to form an emulsion. Whisk in the cilantro or parsley.
5. Combine beans, onions, and garlic, drizzle dressing over, and toss to coat everything.
6. Season to taste with salt and pepper.
7. Marinate in the fridge at least an hour before serving. The longer the beans marinate, the stronger will be the taste. This dish keeps in the refrigerator for up to 4 days.

Variations:
- Use other bean combinations like white beans and red adzuki, or whatever you have on hand.
- Use frozen or BPA (bisphenol-A) free canned garbanzos or kidney beans. You can still get many valuable nutrients from frozen or canned beans.
- Add herbs of your choice for the dressing. For a more pungent flavor, use raw onions and garlic instead of cooked.

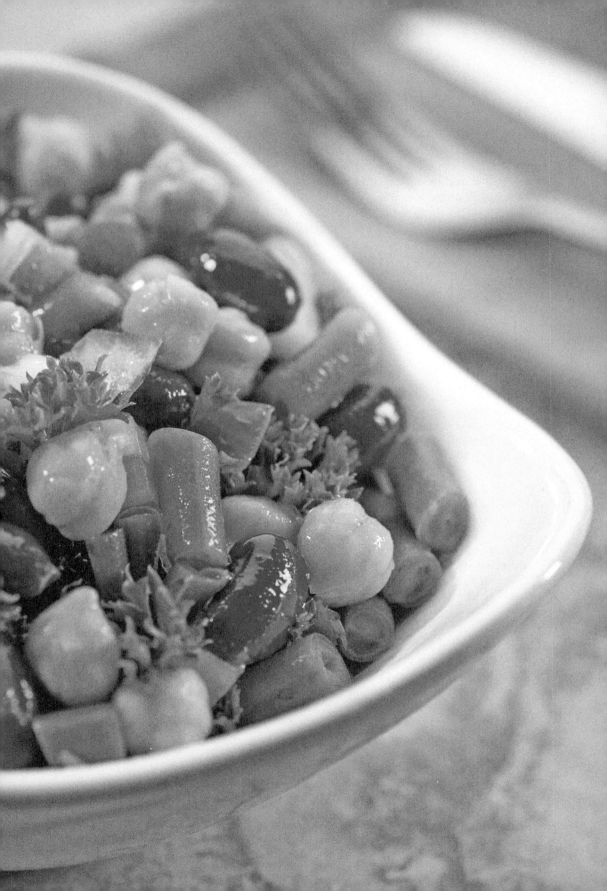

Black Turtle Beans

4 servings

Black beans, also called turtle beans, provide a good texture and are easily used in many dishes. Change the flavor by adding a variety of vegetables and your favorite spices, such as fennel, cumin, savory, or bay leaf, near the end of cooking. For a meatless chili dish, add green and red peppers, tomatoes, and chili peppers. Add more water to prepare a soup.

Ingredients:
1 cup black turtle beans
3 cups filtered or spring water
1-inch piece kombu, soaked 10 minutes
¼ tsp. sea salt per cup of beans
1 cup of fresh yellow corn
Garnish: diced red pepper, chopped parsley

Preparation:
1. Wash beans, cover with water, and soak for 8 hours or overnight.
2. Drain and cover with fresh water, or use another soaking method from this Step.
3. Place beans, water, and soaked kombu in a pot. Bring to a boil without a cover and reduce the flame to simmer.
4. Skim and discard the black foam that floats to the surface. Replace scooped-out water.
5. Cover and cook 60–90 minutes, or until beans are about 90% done. If more water is needed during the cooking time, gently add it along the sides of the pot.
6. Add sea salt and the fresh corn. Shake the pot gently to mix the beans with the juice.
7. Continue cooking until beans are soft and most of the remaining liquid has evaporated.
8. Transfer to a serving dish and garnish. Eat with a grain and vegetable dish.

Variations:
- Add other seasonal vegetables such as chopped carrots.
- Toast the beans in a pan before soaking.
- Pressure-cook beans for 45 minutes, or use timetable of your cooker.
- Use black soybeans instead of black turtle beans.

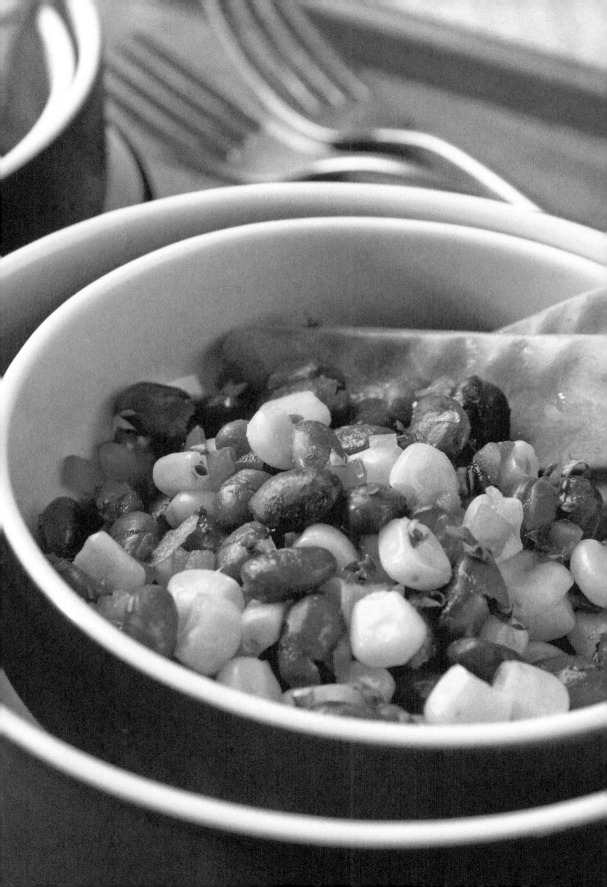

Tempeh Sandwich with Greens and Root Vegetable

4 servings

Tempeh is a fermented whole soybean product, originally from Indonesia, with a rich, nutty flavor. It comes in a square or rectangular block about ½ inch thick. As it has a complete protein profile and ample calcium and isoflavones, it is used regularly in many plant-based cuisines around the world. This dish provides strong energy and is great to eat more often during the fall and winter seasons.

Ingredients:
1 pack tempeh
2–4 tbsp. extra virgin olive oil
3–6 tbsp. tamari
½ tsp. fresh rosemary minced, or ¼ tsp. dried, or to taste (optional)
Filtered or spring water
White daikon root, as needed, finely sliced
Greens like watercress or kale; adjust amounts as needed, sliced

Preparation:
1. Cut tempeh into small strips.
1. Heat the oil and fry the tempeh on both sides till light brown.
1. Place on a paper towel to remove excess oil.
1. Put tempeh in a skillet and add tamari, minced rosemary, and water to cover.
1. Simmer for 20 minutes. Set aside.
2. Wash daikon root with a vegetable brush and slice into thin slices. Steam and set aside.
3. Wash, slice, and steam the greens slightly.
4. To serve as a sandwich, layer daikon and greens between tempeh.

Variations:
• Soak tempeh covered in tamari before using.
• Bake the tempeh for 45 minutes at 375° F instead of frying.
• Prepare it as a spicy dish by adding chili pepper.
• Use a variety of other root vegetables like carrots, turnips, or rutabaga instead of daikon.
• Use herbs like parsley or scallions, and simmer in a broth with miso paste or tahini.
• For a smoky maple flavor dish, simmer tempeh with tamari, smoked sea salt, black pepper, and maple syrup.

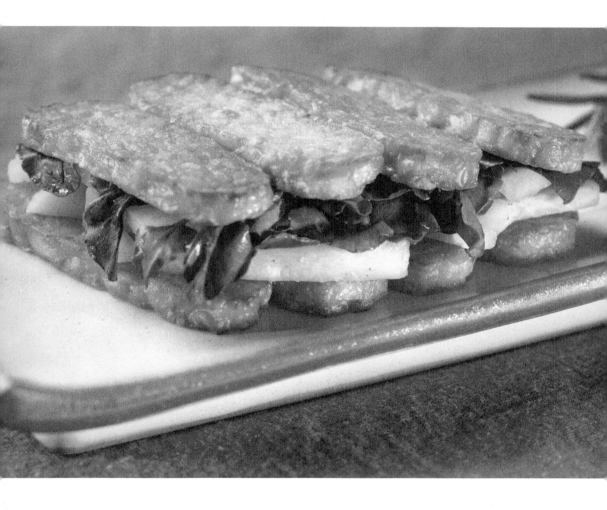

Nori-Wrapped Tofu with Miso

4 servings

This dish combines the power of three wonderful foods. Tofu is a high-protein soybean product and is easy to digest. Miso is a fermented food that helps with digestion. Nori sea vegetable is packed with minerals and other nutrients.

__Ingredients:__
16-ounce pack hard tofu, rinsed and drained well
2 tsp. miso, flavor of your choice, to spread on the inside of the tofu slices
Thinly sliced carrots, steamed, to yield 8–10 pieces, or as needed
Watercress or other greens, 8–10 pieces, or as needed
2 sheets toasted nori sea vegetable, cut into ½-inch strips
Oil for baking dish
2–4 tbsp. rice miso diluted with warm water, to cover tofu

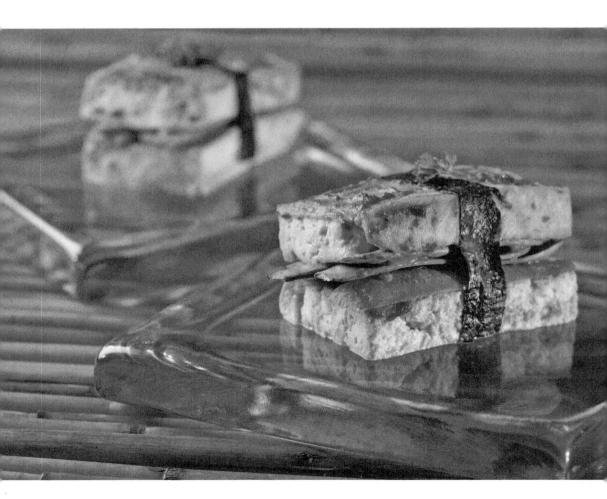

Preparation:

1. Preheat oven to 375° F.
2. Cut the tofu into ½-inch slices starting at the short end, and then halve the long way.
3. Spread miso on one side of a slice of tofu, add steamed carrot slices and watercress or other greens, and put a second slice of tofu on top.
4. Wrap a small strip of nori around both pieces and place into an oiled 8 x 8 baking dish. Repeat till all the tofu slices are used.
5. Mix warm water and miso in a separate bowl, and pour over the tofu in the baking dish.
6. Cover dish with parchment paper and bake at 375° F for about 30 minutes.
7. Serve two "sandwiches" per person, with a grain dish and a fresh green salad on the side.

Variations:

- Place slightly cooked slices of daikon in between the tofu pieces.
- Marinate tofu slices in a 1-to-1 tamari/water mixture ½–1 hour before baking (for a saltier taste) to cover. Turn, if needed, to marinate on both sides.

Smoky Black-Peppered Seared Green Beans

2–4 side servings

Smoked sea salt has been a favorite in the seasoning trade since around the eighth century. It is said that the Vikings infused crystal sea salt with this flavor by smoking it over aromatic wood fires.

Ingredients:

1 lb. green beans with ends removed
2 tbsp. toasted sesame oil
1 tsp. smoked sea salt
¾ tsp. coarse-ground black pepper
1/3 cup sliced almonds
1 tbsp. fresh lemon juice

Preparation:

1. Wash green beans, drain well, and cut into 2–3" pieces.
2. Heat large cast iron skillet until just too hot to touch. Add oil and spread evenly across skillet.
3. Add green beans and cook for 2–3 minutes, tossing often. Cooking time will vary slightly depending on the size and freshness of the green beans.
4. Add smoky sea salt, black pepper, and sliced almonds. Cook for another 2–3 minutes, tossing often and adjusting heat if necessary, so as not to burn them.
5. Beans and almonds should be slightly blackened.
6. Add lemon juice, turn off heat, and let lemon juice absorb.
7. Remove from skillet immediately and serve.

Variations:

- If smoked sea salt is not available, use regular sea salt and more black pepper.
- Experiment with your favorite spices for this dish.

Sprouted Mung Bean Salad with Lemon Dressing

4 servings

Sprouting beans or seeds increases their nutritional value tenfold. Get sprouts at the store, or enjoy how plant life unfolds in your kitchen. It's easy to sprout them yourself, and kids love helping out too. All you need are the beans, a Mason jar with a screen and lid, filtered or spring water, a clean kitchen, and a few days' time.

Ingredients:
1 cup mung bean sprouts, purchased or home-sprouted
Filtered or spring water, room temperature
1 bag red radishes, cleaned, halved, and finely sliced
3 stems scallions, sliced
2 sticks celery, sliced
1 medium carrot, shredded
1 cup parsley, minced
1 cup chickpeas, cooked or sprouted

Dressing:
Juice of one lemon plus lemon zest, or to taste
Pinch sea salt or Himalayan salt
¼ tsp. dulse sea vegetable flakes (optional)
3 tsp. flax oil or extra virgin olive oil (optional)

Preparation:
1. Home-sprouted: Start 2–3 days ahead of time:
2. Rinse about ¼ cup beans in room-temperature water and drain.
3. Put beans in Mason jar and secure its screen using the ring portion of the lid.
4. Four times a day, swirl beans in room temperature water and drain again. Prop the inverted jar at an angle in sink or bowl to remove all water each time.
5. When sprouts are about ¼ inch long, they are ready to eat.
6. Assembly:
7. In a large bowl, mix sprouts, chickpeas, all vegetables, and the dressing, and let marinate for 1 hour. Before serving, drizzle with oil, if using, and mix lightly.
8. Serve as a side dish with grains and steamed vegetables.

Variations:
- Use a variety of other sprouts like alfalfa, amaranth, broccoli, or mustard.
- Press the vegetables with sea salt in a pickle press or a large glass bowl with a plate and a weight on top for one hour before adding the sprouts.
- Use cooked beans instead of sprouted.

Healthy Breakfast or Anytime Bean Dishes

Refried Black Bean Burrito

4 servings

This burrito is great for breakfast, or it can be a healthy meal for anytime or on the go. The bean-spice mixture and the salsa can be prepared in advance and kept in the refrigerator for up to three days.

Ingredients:

2 cups cooked black (turtle) beans
1 tsp. light sesame oil or rice bran oil
Spice blend ingredients:
¼ tsp. sea salt
¾ tsp. ground cumin
¾ tsp. ground oregano
1/8 tsp. garlic powder
Salsa ingredients—equal amounts of:
Diced cucumber
Finely diced red onions
Cooked corn
Minced cilantro
Pinch sea salt
Zest and juice of 1 lemon, or to taste
4 nine-inch whole yellow corn tortillas
2 cups fresh salad greens or cooked greens, sliced

Preparation:

1. Add spice blend ingredients to taste to the beans, and mash thoroughly with a fork.
2. Heat oil in a skillet and add spiced beans, stirring them until they are heated.
3. Use another cast iron skillet to heat each tortilla. Remove quickly.
4. Spread ¼ cup of warmed bean mixture evenly onto each heated tortilla. Leave a 1-inch border.
5. Heat salsa lightly (optional). Ladle about 1 tbsp. salsa over beans.
6. Top with greens.
7. Roll up the tortilla, making sure all edges are folded in.
8. Enjoy as a full light meal with a cup of hot tea.

Variations:

- Use other beans, like navy, pinto, adzuki, kidney, or garbanzo.
- Add cooked grains to the spread before adding the salsa.
- Use other vegetables in the salsa, or add fruits like mango.

Scrambled Tofu

Included in the Vegan Mock Bacon Condiment (Photo in Step 8, page 159)

4 servings

A classic. Scrambled tofu is a great breakfast, brunch, or anytime dish that easily replaces scrambled eggs. Serve it with lightly toasted bread and a good cup of kukicha or green tea.

Ingredients:

1 cake soft tofu
1 tsp. light sesame oil or water
1–2 tbsp. tamari, to taste
1/4 tsp. peeled ginger, grated
1 clove garlic, grated (optional)
2 tsp. scallion greens, cut into thin slices
Garnish: toasted nori, cut into thin strips (optional)

Preparation:

1. Remove tofu from package and rinse. Towel dry.
2. Heat a stainless steel or cast iron skillet, add oil or water, and crumble the tofu into it.
3. Stir in tamari; add ginger, garlic (if using), and scallions. Cover and simmer 5 minutes.
4. Garnish with finely cut strips of nori sea vegetable.
5. Eat with a side of whole grain bread or with cooked grains and vegetables.
6. Or wrap in a warm tortilla of your choice for a breakfast taco.

Variations:

- Add 2 cups of finely cut vegetables of your choice. Choose yellow corn, broccoli, onions, carrots, daikon radish, etc.
- Add spices and seasonings like turmeric or chili.
- Grate mochi over the scrambled tofu and bake in a cast iron skillet, 5 minutes at 350° F.
- Use blue or white corn, whole rice, or sprouted grain tortillas.
- Use smaller tortilla sizes to serve more people.
- *Gluten Advice:* Whole-wheat tortillas contain gluten—use corn instead.

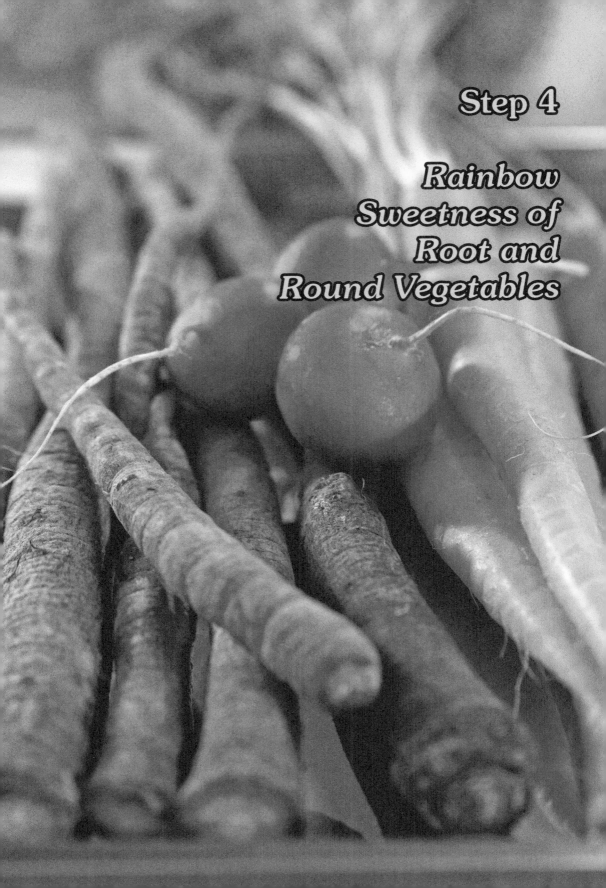

Step 4 introduces a wide variety of root and round vegetables, with a wonderful kaleidoscope of colors and shapes, into your cooking repertoire. These vegetables are high in vitamins and minerals and provide dietary fiber, which is good for digestion.

Most have a naturally sweet flavor, which helps to reduce the need for eating too many sweets. Winter squashes, onions, and carrots also soothe the internal organs and energize the mind. Opt to include several servings of these nutrient-dense vegetables into your daily meals of greens, grains, and beans as a valuable addition to balance your plate.

History and Names of Some Root and Round Vegetables

Most root and round vegetables have a long history as cultivated vegetables enjoyed in many cultures.[45]

Root Vegetables

Root vegetables are the starchy tubers or taproots of plants. They grow under the earth, where the plant concentrates its energy and nourishment. They provide strong downward (yang) energy, in contrast to the green leafy vegetables, which provide more upward energy (yin).

You are certainly familiar with carrots, potatoes, and onions—root vegetables you already use often in your kitchen. We encourage you to try other delicious and nourishing roots, such as burdock, parsnip, ginger root, celery root, rutabaga, yams, sweet potatoes, turnips, parsnips, red radishes, white radish (daikon), and black radish. One root vegetable, the lotus root, rows in water. Some cultivated root vegetables, like white daikon and red radishes, are mostly known for their tasty roots, yet they also provide nourishing greens, thus allowing us to eat the whole plant.

Other root vegetables, like dandelion (yes, you can eat the roots), are very long and narrow, and if you find them growing in a natural garden that is chemical-free and unsprayed, you can dig them out and eat them. These roots can be tenacious, so it may require a lot of digging. Dandelion roots are also often sold dried as teas. The young dandelion greens are a tasty wild addition to your early spring meals, and you can also find them in many markets. Pick the yellow dandelion flowers too, as these are edible when in season.

Burdock root is native to northern China and Siberia and has been cultivated, mostly in Japan, since the tenth century, where it is called *gobo,* and is used in making *kimpira,* a traditional Japanese dish. In Europe and the US, it grows wild on forest ways, and thus it is the perfect survival food. Learn how to recognize wild burdock during your nature walks by its very large, roundish green leaves. These leaves are not edible—all the available nourishment for humans in burdock is in the long brown roots. You can dig out this wild growing root, if you are so inclined, in its first or second growing season. Cultivated burdock root, dandelion root, and lotus root are available at Asian markets, natural food stores, or online.

Turnips have been used as a staple vegetable in Europe and Asia since prehistoric times. Also called *timpsula* by the Lakota Sioux, turnips were for centuries the most important wild food gathered by the Native American peoples.[46] They grew in prairies throughout the Great Plains from Saskatchewan to north Texas. You can still find some in Dakota grasslands that have not been cultivated or heavily foraged. The Native American "fry bread" was historically made with dried wild turnip flour. Nowadays, cultivated turnips are eaten in stews, roasted, boiled, or mashed.

Onions have been an important part of our diet since the beginning of civilization. They grow wild on every continent, though their cultivation probably began in Asia around 3500 BC. Onions are one of the few foods that can be stored during the winter without refrigeration. They belong to the Allium genus of bulb-shaped plants, which also includes scallions, chives, garlic, and leeks.

The edible carrot was cultivated in Afghanistan as far back as 5,000 years ago. Purple carrots can be seen in temple drawings of Egypt from 2000 BC, and carrot seeds were found in the crypts of pharaohs. Later, many colorful varieties were found in Asia and Europe. The history of carrots and parsnips is intertwined, probably because of their similar shapes and colors.[47]

Radishes have been domesticated in Europe since pre-Roman times and are grown and consumed throughout the world. You can find numerous varieties in different sizes and colors. The most familiar are the small round red ones, and daikon, a cylindrical white radish that may be as long as 20 inches. Daikon was introduced to Asia around 500 BC.[48]

Round Vegetables

Squashes or pumpkins have been found in the wild for over 10,000 years in North and Central America. Native Americans even buried them with their dead to provide them nourishment on their final journey. The butternut squash, which is related to the pumpkin, was not generally eaten until the nineteenth century, but is now the most widely grown winter squash. There are numerous varieties of squash available, many with meaty qualities and mildly sweet tastes. The Japanese Hokkaido pumpkin is often used in the macrobiotic cuisine because of its rich, concentrated flavor.[49]

During the autumn harvest season, you can find a wide variety of hard-skinned squashes like acorn, butternut, buttercup, Hubbard, orange pumpkin, and Hokkaido pumpkin. These squashes and pumpkins are part of the gourd family, and you can use them in soups, desserts, as main dishes, or as decoration.

During the summer months, you can choose from a variety of summer squashes like zucchini or pattypan. These enjoyable delights are easy to cut and steam, compared to their stronger-tasting autumn relatives with their harder skins. Summer squashes have a light yin energy compared to fall squashes, which are more yang.

Vegetables with different appearances like red and green cabbage, kale, kohlrabi, cauliflower, broccoli, and Brussels sprouts are all members of the same species, *Brassica oleracea*, known as the cruciferous vegetables, and each has developed via small changes over time.[50] The first wild ancestor of the cabbage plant was eaten about 7,000 years ago in the Mediterranean region of Europe. We use cruciferous vegetables in preparing many delicious dishes.

Mushrooms belong to the kingdom of fungi and are not necessarily round vegetables, but we decided to add them to this vegetables list. The most commonly used mushrooms in the macrobiotic kitchen are the *shiitake* (in dried form), as these provide the best flavor, when rehydrated, and are known for their healing properties. There are many other edible mushrooms, like the wild-harvested truffle or the cultivated white button mushroom. The *maitake* (dancing mushroom), *reishi* (spiritual mushroom), *kikurage* (tree mushroom), and *saru-no-koshikake* (stool for monkey) are grown in the high mountains and on high trees. They are used as special remedies, though only a small volume can be used in cooking and baking or in dried powder form. They can add nutritional value and wonderful flavors to your dishes and can be enjoyed from time to time.

A Rainbow Color Nutrient Guide

You can find vegetables in many colors, from red (yang), to many in between, to white (yin). Use the vibrant colors of vegetables and fruits as your guide in your kitchen to attract the benefits of the powerful nutrients each of these color families can provide.[51]

Green

Green vegetables are a great source of nutrients, including folate, minerals, fiber, and antioxidants. Some greens can protect against cataracts and macular degeneration and can reduce cancer risks. For more information on green leafy vegetables, read Step 1.

Orange and Yellow

Carrots, sweet potatoes, orange pumpkins and squashes (as well as oranges, apricots, and mangoes) provide beta-carotene, which boosts the immune system, and vitamin C and folate, which reduce the risk of heart disease. These vegetables are often high in potassium too. Beta-carotene, lutein, and zeaxanthin all are powerful antioxidants that seem to play a role in blocking early stages of cancer. Orange vegetables are easy to include in stir-fries and stews and are delicious simply oven-roasted with a drizzle of olive oil and perhaps some herbs.

Red

Red radishes, red beets, red cabbages, red onions, red chili peppers (and also red fruits like strawberries, raspberries, and pomegranates) contain lycopene, the antioxidant that helps protect against heart disease and some types of cancer, mainly prostate cancer.

Blue and Purple

Red cabbage, red onions, and beets (as well as blueberries, purple grapes, and plums) get their color from anthocyanin, a phytochemical that protects against carcinogens and may help prevent heart disease.

White

The white hues of onions, garlic, cauliflower, and some other vegetables signify allicin, which can help lower cholesterol and blood pressure. White daikon radish is abundant in digestive enzymes similar to those found in the human digestive tract.

Seasonal Reflections - When to Eat Your Vegetables

Don't you love the idea of eating what is grown locally and in season? Fresh foods harvested and eaten at their nutritional peak taste so delicious and provide you with exceptional energy. When you consume more locally grown foods from your garden or other nearby sources, you also reduce the carbon footprint of your lifestyle. Use the chart below to create root and round vegetable dishes that are energetically supportive for the season.

Spring	Summer	Late Summer	Autumn	Winter
Kohlrabi Red round radishes Small white radishes Spring onions Young small carrots	Cucumber Early carrots Fennel Garlic Pattypan squash Peppers Tomatoes Zucchini	Eggplant Parsnip Pumpkin Squash Sweet potato Turnip Yam	Artichokes Brussels sprouts Cabbage Cauliflower Celery root Daikon Dandelion root Ginger Long carrots Lotus root Mushrooms Onion Savoy cabbage Squash (fall) Shiitake White radish	Beet root Black radish Brussels sprouts Burdock Chicory root Water chestnut

Health Benefits of Root and Round Vegetables

Pros:

- Raw daikon radish helps to break down animal foods like meat, dairy, and eggs. Use it immediately after you grate it, as after 30 minutes nearly 50 percent of its enzymes are lost. For the grated daikon recipe, see Step 10.
- Many root and round vegetables, like carrots, onions, parsnips, rutabaga, cabbage, and winter squashes, have a naturally sweet taste when properly cooked. Rather than depending on processed sugar for sweets, make these your healthy and delicious first choices.
- Squashes, onions, and cabbage are beneficial for supporting and softening pancreas, spleen, and stomach energy, and can help to stabilize blood sugar levels. Prepare a broth, drinks, or specialty dishes with these vegetables to satisfy your sweet tooth and reduce sugar cravings.
- Cruciferous vegetables such as cabbage, Brussels sprouts, and cauliflower contain antioxidants and other phytonutrients that reduce cancer risk.
- Burdock root (gobo) and its extracts are valued for blood purification, arthritis relief, and skin disease prevention, destruction of bacteria and fungus, and cancer fighting. Burdock is also said to be a glycemic index regulator, which means it helps to slow down the dumping of sugars into the system. Burdock is one of the ingredients in Essiac, a tea based on an Ojibwa formula that is used as an immune enhancer and for some kinds of cancer.
- Onions lower cholesterol and contain antioxidants that help block cancer. Garlic has healing properties and is said to clean the blood. It is used in many cuisines to balance heavy meat or dairy dishes. Because of its strong smell that stays with

you for a while, use it as an optional choice in your dishes. Energetically it has a yin character, and it is not preferred during meditation.

Cons:

- Since some of these round vegetables also contain starch, overeating them could result in weight gain. Consider them in the context of your starch intake when you are on a weight-loss diet, and choose to eat more green leafy vegetables instead. Yet daikon root, burdock root, and lotus roots are helpful to slim down.
- The nightshade plants—potatoes, tomatoes, bell peppers, and eggplants (and tobacco)—are alkaloids, and many alkaloids are toxic. These vegetables are better used only seldom in your macrobiotic kitchen. Eating these often, even within their growing season, could make you feel weak. They are very cooling, with extreme yin energy, and thus could take your vigor. Anecdotal evidence suggests that eating nightshades can aggravate arthritis tendencies, and increased pain has been experienced when they are eaten regularly. In general, if a person finds that certain foods make them feel ill or unhealthy, it makes sense to avoid them.

Way of Life Inspirations

- If you are out of alignment because of having "too many things on your plate," take a deep breath and make a good meal instead. Basic life-sustaining activities, like eating good, whole, healthy foods, should take priority over computer games or watching TV, or even more productive pursuits (if done to excess).
- Involve the family in making changes that are good for their health. Get out the carrots and radishes and make a delicious dish. Your body and mind will thank you for it.
- Cultivate pleasant physical activities to recharge your energy. Take daily outside walks or use a bicycle whenever you can instead of driving. Look into contemplative movement like tai chi, qigong, or yoga that will help keep you fit.
- Nurture honest and open relationships that feed your soul. Take a relaxed and moderate position in conflict situations, and foster peace of mind. When difficulties arise, clear them up as soon as possible. Don't carry them around for too long.
- Focus on meaningful relaxation to calm and nourish your spirit and mood. Remember to take deep breaths during the day, and stretch often. Spend time in nature, go into the forest, read a good book, or plant a garden.

Macrobiotic Yin and Yang Vegetable Cooking Guide

To master the art of macrobiotic cooking, seasonal balance is important. As much as possible, use freshly bought, organically grown seasonal vegetables, and choose cooking techniques well suited for the season. In the hotter months (yang), use the more yin foods that grow during that time, and vice versa—in the winter (yin), choose more yang winter vegetables.

These are important characteristics that make macrobiotic cooking different from other regimens. After cooking for several seasons, you will have mastered your new kitchen habits. You will be in tune with your own needs, and creating your own recipes will become second nature. Root and round vegetables combine well with bean or grain dishes and can offer additional ways to explore contracting (yang) or expanding (yin) energy in your meals.

Vegetable Shapes below the Earth

Looking at vegetable shapes, we find that long roots like carrots have a more concentrated energy (yang) compared to the roundish roots like the onions, which have more expansive (yin) energy. The long and slender burdock has the most yang energy compared to other root vegetables. It can strengthen your concentration and provide an energetic feeling of being grounded because of its downward yang energy.

Vegetable Shapes above the Earth

Shapes also vary among the vegetables growing on top of the earth. Some are rounder; some are slender or oblong. But the shape comparison is just the opposite from the root vegetables. Top-growing round vegetables present yang energy, and top-growing slender or oblong shapes have a more yin energy.

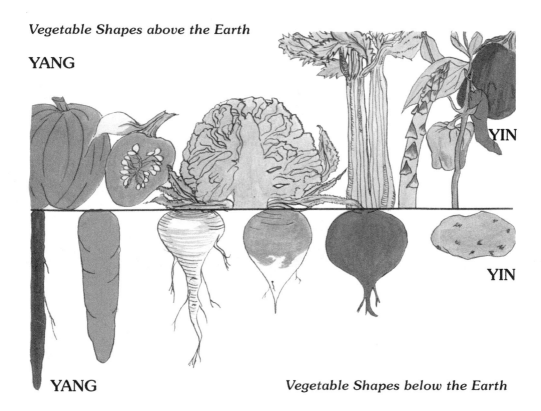

Vegetable Shapes above the Earth

YANG

YIN

YIN

YANG

Vegetable Shapes below the Earth

Preparing Vegetables

Wash the vegetables thoroughly with a brush. Remove any blemishes, bruises, fine rootlets, or eyes with a peeler or skinning knife. Many organic root and round vegetables don't need to be peeled. Remove the skin only if the vegetables are chemically sprayed or waxed. Many of the nutrients are found right under the skin. Some of the roots or rounds can also be cooked or baked whole with the skin attached and peeled afterwards, if needed.

   Note about soup stocks: If your recipe calls for peeling the skin, you can use most of the organic vegetable peels to make a delicious soup stock. Boil them in water for about one hour and use in soups, stews, or other dishes.

Vegetable Cutting Styles

It is important to eat more vegetables, regardless of the cutting style you use. However, cutting styles can be yin or yang and influence the cooking time and thus the quality of the result. Do not be discouraged from eating vegetables while you are learning new cutting styles in the recipes. Use good quality knives, and it is fine to make use of a mandolin or some other kitchen device to achieve the styles you need.

   Smaller cutting techniques like matchstick (julienne), mincing, or fine dicing are yang methods. Slicing a root vegetable (yang) in a matchstick style (yang) results in a concentrated yang dish. You can use this combination if, for instance, a person needs more concentrated energy in a winter month (yin), or as a substitute for an animal dish (yang), or to balance the quality of the meal.

   Using larger chunks is a yin cutting style. When you cut larger chunks (yin) of a root vegetable (yang), the dish is more balanced. Cutting a green leafy vegetable (yin) in a larger style (yin) creates an expanding quality. Use this preparation in the hot

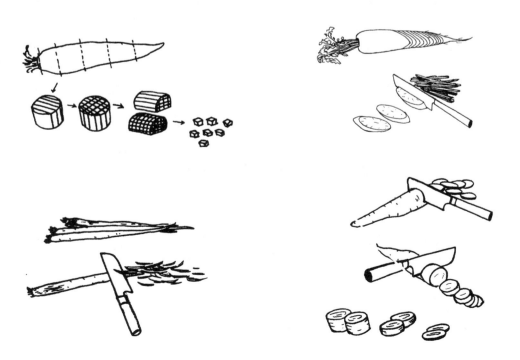

summer season (yang), for relaxing energy (yin), or to balance the yang quality of a meal. A matchstick cutting style (yang) for a green vegetable (yin) can also yield a more balanced dish.

Seasonings

The seasonings of your food will also influence the quality of the dish. For instance, sea salt or tamari (yang) brings out a different quality of the food than vinegar (yin). Garnish all of your cooked dishes (yang) using fresh and raw herbs (yin) such as spring onions, scallions, coriander leaves, parsley, or basil, as these are all rich sources of vitamins, including vitamin C.

Cooking Temperatures

Your cooking temperatures can help you balance your energy during each season. Adding heat to your food through cooking is considered yang, and using raw foods or less heat is considered yin. Use less heat in summer season, which is a yang energy season, and more heat in winter cooking, which is a more yin energy season. A general way of cooking a vegetable dish in any season is brief steaming or boiling to preserve most of the nutrients. In summer you can choose to prepare, in addition, more raw salads (yin) or lightly short-time fermented foods. In the colder winter seasons (yin), in addition, use more yang preparations like pressure-cooking or baking, dried foods, or long-time fermented foods.

Cooking Times

You can also influence the yin and yang quality of the food by using a variety of cooking times—long, short, and raw—depending on the season and your needs. Longer cooking time produces a stronger dish (yang), whereas short time cooking produces a lighter dish (yin). Use less time in the summer season, which is a yang energy season, and more time in winter cooking, which is a more yin energy season. When cooking vegetables for a longer time, heat-sensitive nutrients like vitamin C are lost, whereas other nutrients, like beta-carotene, become more readily available through cooking.

Storing Vegetables

Fresh vegetables are best washed and then stored in a cool place. This way they are easy to use when you need them.

Some vegetables can be dried and then stored. Dried food is considered more yang than the same food in its fresh state. Just rehydrate dried foods by soaking them in water when you want to cook them. Macrobiotic dried-vegetable favorites like daikon, lotus root, burdock, and dandelion root add interesting textures and variations to your meals. Use more dried vegetables (yang) in the colder seasons (yin) to balance your plate. You can dry vegetables yourself—hang-dry them, or use a dehydrator. You can also buy already dried vegetables and herbs in grocery stores, or order online.

Preserving Vegetables

Root and round vegetables also preserve well as pickled or fermented foods. Stock up on sauerkraut and umeboshi plums. When eaten daily in small amounts, raw fermented foods aid digestion and provide vitamins and enzymes. For further information and recipes, see Step 5.

Freezing Vegetables

When fresh vegetables are not available, have some in your freezer. You can always buy them, but you can also blanch and then freeze them yourself when in season. Frozen vegetables are acceptable solutions, especially for frequent travelers, working parents, or single eaters who need instant, good-quality nourishment. Frozen foods are considered more yin than fresh. They are easy to toss into a pan or steam for a few minutes (not too long, as they easily get mushy). Frozen vegetables should not, however, completely replace fresh vegetables.

Cooking for Wellness

When you are cooking for wellness, you need to be aware of ingredients and methods that speak directly to the issue at hand. See Step 10 – *Kitchen Remedies, Tonics, and Therapies* on how to prepare a few specialty dishes with fresh or dried vegetables. Get advice from your health-care provider and nutritionist on which foods best support your needs.

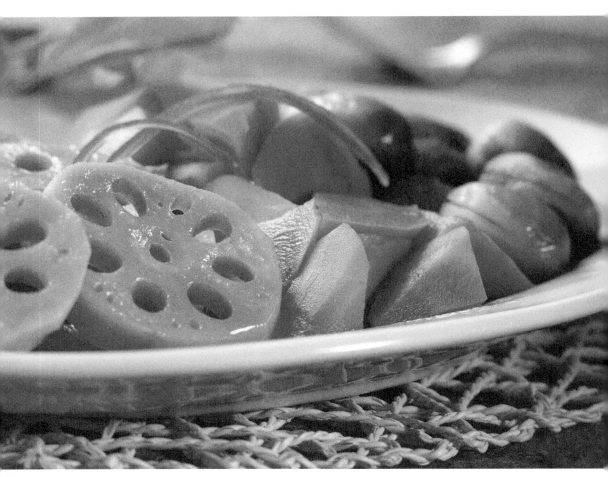

Recipes for Root and Round Vegetables

Seasonal Nishime Cooking Style – Waterless Cooking

Adjustable servings

Nishime cooking, or waterless cooking is a braising method that means cooking large chunks of vegetables in very little water over low heat for a longer time in a sturdy pot. This produces strong and radiant energy and a deep sweetness. Classic nishime style usually calls for a combination of three or five vegetables, but you can include more, or even use just one.

Ingredients:

Allow a handful of each seasonal vegetable per person:
Autumn/Winter: Carrot/burdock/lotus root, or burdock/lotus root/daikon
Autumn: Squash, cabbage, onion, daikon, shiitake mushrooms
Late summer: parsnip, pumpkin, turnip
Spring: kohlrabi, early carrots
1-inch piece kombu sea vegetable
Filtered or spring water to half cover the vegetables
Sprinkles of sea salt
Tamari to taste (optional)

Preparation:

1. Scrub and, if not organic, peel vegetables. Cut into large bite-size pieces.
2. Soak kombu in water for 10 minutes. Remove.
3. Place kombu at the bottom of a heavy pot and layer the vegetables, or place them in sections around the pot.
4. Add one to two inches of water to half cover the vegetables. (Optional: use the kombu soaking water.)
5. Add sprinkles of sea salt and cover the pot with a heavy lid.
6. Bring to a boil to generate steam, then lower the heat and simmer till just about done. If the water evaporates too quickly during the cooking, add more water.
7. Add the tamari, if using, and toss the pot gently—with the lid on.
8. Continue to simmer on low 2–4 minutes. Total cooking time is 15–20 minutes or less, depending on the vegetables you are using.
9. Remove the lid, turn off the flame, and let the vegetables breathe for about two minutes.
10. Serve, including any remaining liquid along with the vegetables.
11. This dish complements a quick steamed green vegetable and a grain dish with beans.

Variations:

- This cooking style is good to use with root vegetables, but some top-growing vegetables like squashes, cabbage, and even mushrooms also taste good this way.
- In the late summer, when outside energies are still warm, prepare this dish using seasonal vegetables and serve about twice per week.
- In the autumn and winter, when outside conditions are cold, prepare it with seasonal vegetables every other day.

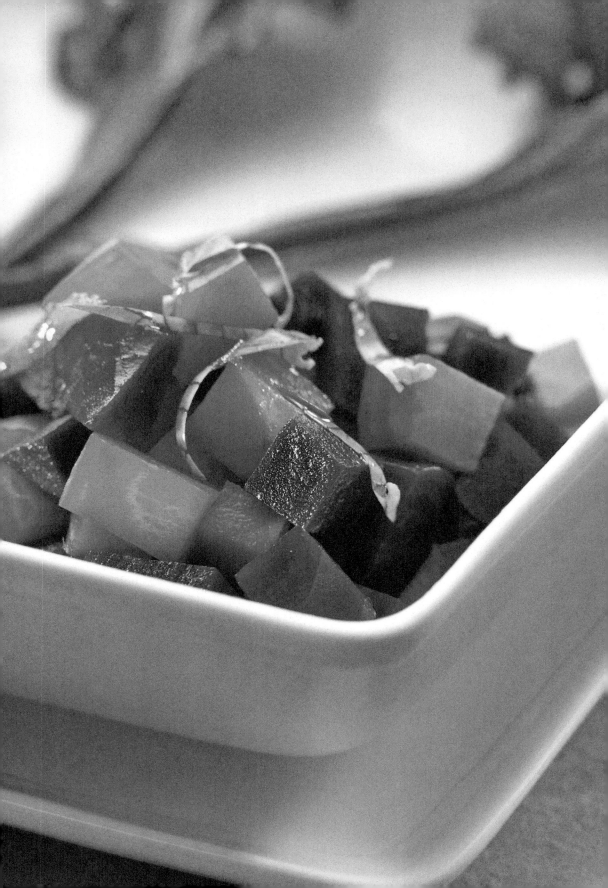

Braised Red Beets

3 sides, or serve as appetizer

Beets are outstanding for their nutritional density. The beet is a yin-shape round root vegetable. In summer or winter, beets provide a colorful addition to your meals. Because beets lose their color easily and tend to dye everything they come in contact with, cutting them on a plastic board or under running water will allow you to wash away any stains immediately.

Ingredients:

1½ pounds red beets
Filtered or spring water
¼ tsp. sea salt
1 tbsp. umeboshi vinegar, or to taste
1 tsp. brown rice syrup (optional)

Dressing:

1 shallot, minced, raw, or steamed (optional)
¼ tsp. sea salt, or to taste
1 tbsp. lemon zest, minced
Extra virgin olive oil, to taste

Parsley, minced

Preparation:

1. Wash and dice the beets. Place them in pot and half-cover with water.
2. Add sea salt and bring to a boil. Simmer for about 20 minutes or until soft.
3. Drain, reserving liquid, and put into a serving bowl.
4. Heat reserved liquid. Add vinegar and (optional) syrup and simmer, stirring occasionally to reduce liquid.
5. Remove from heat and add shallots, sea salt, and lemon zest. Toss with beets. Let marinate for about ½ hour before serving (optional).
6. Serve with drizzle of extra virgin olive oil and minced parsley.

Variations:

• In the summer, cool down beets in the refrigerator and serve chilled.
• Use red wine vinegar instead of umeboshi vinegar.
• Add toasted nuts or seeds to the mix.
• Sidestep roasting beets, as most nutrients are lost.

White Daikon Radish with Sea Vegetables and Shiitake Mushroom
–A Macrobiotic Cleansing Dish

3–4 servings

The white daikon radish has enzymatic properties that help to digest your food, especially fat, and cleanse your blood. Eat it raw and add it to pressed salads or grated as a garnish for fried dishes. Boil, steam, or roast it alone or with other vegetables. Dried or dehydrated white daikon radish tastes sweet and has concentrated healing properties. For a deep cleansing, make this recipe a couple of times per month.

Ingredients:

2-inch piece kombu sea vegetable
1–2 dried shiitake mushrooms
1–2 cups fresh white daikon radish, or ½ cup dried white daikon radish
1 tsp. tamari, or to taste
Filtered or spring water

Preparation:

1. Cover kombu and dried shiitake with water and soak for about 10 minutes.
2. Slice kombu into ¼-inch pieces and place at the bottom of a heavy pot with a lid.
3. Remove tip of stem from soaked shiitake, slice into small pieces, and place on top of the kombu.
4. If using dried daikon, soak covered with water for 10 minutes. Drain and slice, and layer on top of the mushrooms.
5. If using fresh daikon, wash, scrub, and cut into 1-inch big round pieces and layer on top.
6. Use the kombu and shiitake soaking water and add fresh water to half cover the vegetables. (If using dried daikon, add the soaking water if it has a light color.)
7. Add tamari, bring to a quick boil, and then lower the flame and cover the pot.
8. Simmer 30–40 minutes or until the vegetables are soft. Cook away the excess liquid. Reseason with tamari, if needed.

Variations:

• Try round red radishes instead of daikon and use fresh shiitake instead of dried for a lighter cleanse.

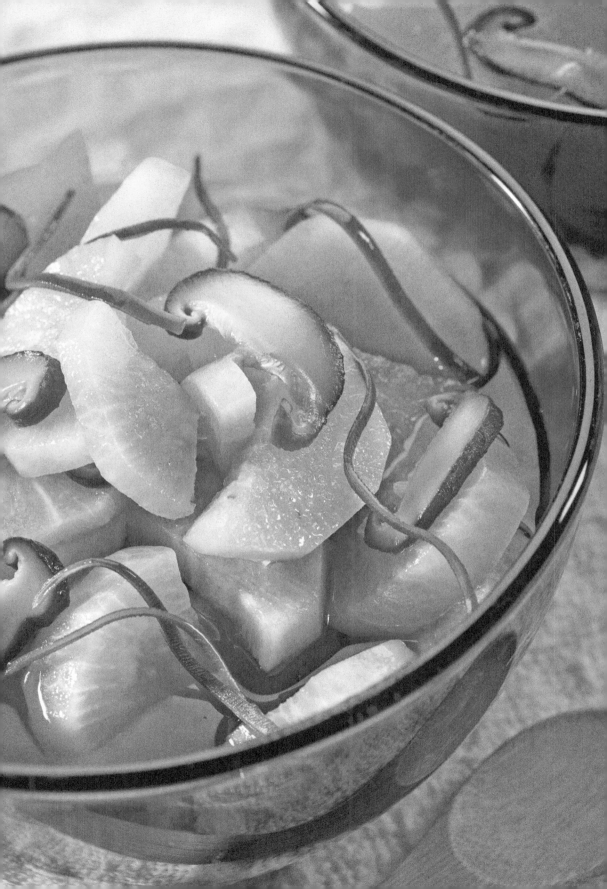

Mashed Potato-Style Parsnips with Cauliflower

(Photo includes the Mushroom-Onion Sauce with Tamari and Ginger from Step 8, p. 160)

4–6 servings

Parsnips, with their distinct flavor, give this dish a special quality you might like to try for comfort food instead of your usual mashed potatoes. Cauliflower is high in nutrients like vitamin C, but is low in calories and thus a great food for healthy weight control. Eat as is or serve with the *Mushroom Onion Sauce with Tamari and Ginger* from Step 8.

Ingredients:

1½ lbs. parsnip
1 small head of cauliflower, cut into small florets
Pinch sea salt
½ cup unsweetened non-dairy milk, warmed
1 tbsp. extra virgin olive oil, or to taste
Sea salt and freshly ground black pepper, to taste
Filtered or spring water

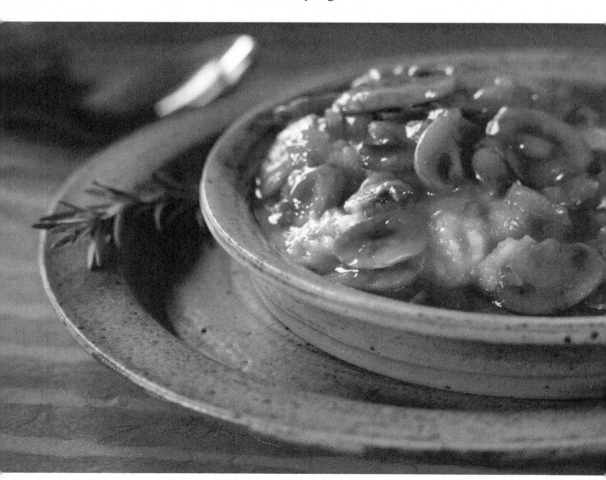

Preparation:

1. Wash and scrub the parsnips. Remove skin to achieve a smoother texture when mashing (optional), and cut into ½–1-inch chunks.
2. Place the parsnips and the florets of cauliflower into a large saucepan.
3. Half cover with water, add a pinch of sea salt, bring to a boil, and simmer gently, about 12 minutes, or until all is very tender.
4. Drain well and mash in a suribachi, adding just enough non-dairy milk to get the texture you prefer. Leave a few lumps if you like. (Instead of a suribachi, use a food mill or power hand blender if you prefer a smoother texture.)
5. Drizzle in the olive oil, season with sea salt and pepper to taste, and mix.

Variations:

- Use other root vegetables like turnips or carrots and mash them by themselves or in combination with other root or round vegetables.
- Mash up a cooked squash for a sweeter sensation.
- Use unsweetened plain soymilk, almond milk, or rice milk.
- Add ¼ tsp. nutmeg.
- Try adding about 1 tsp. chickpea miso.

Red Cabbage Sautéed with Red Apples

6 servings

This dish is a childhood favorite of mine. In European cuisine, we often use wine to enhance the flavor of a dish. Match the color of the cabbage with the color of the apple and the wine. Make this dish with green cabbage, green apples and white wine.

Ingredients:

1 tbsp. extra virgin olive oil
1 medium onion, diced (optional)
1 medium red apple, cored and diced
1 small red cabbage, cored and sliced finely
1 tsp. sea salt
1 tsp. fresh grated or dried garlic (optional)
1 cup red wine, or to taste (optional)
Filtered or spring water

Preparation:

1. Heat oil in a stainless steel pot.
2. Add onions (if using), then apple, and then cabbage, stirring after each addition. Add the sea salt, garlic, and red wine (if using), or water, and mix again.
3. Bring to a boil, cover, and simmer for about 10 minutes or until cabbage is soft and tasty.
4. Serve as a side dish with whole grains and a bean dish.

Variations:

- Use a few drops of vinegar (red wine or umeboshi) instead of 1 cup of red wine for a tangier taste.

Stuffed Pumpkin–A Possible Holiday Affair

Note: Photo *Savory Wild Rice with Sautéed Vegetables–A Possible Holiday Stuffing* from Step 2, p. 51 includes the pumpkin

2–3 entrée servings

Make this dish anytime, or use it as a vegan entrée during holidays. Make it instead of the usual holiday stuffed turkey that is commonly eaten in North America. Assemble with the *Savory Wild Rice with Sautéed Vegetables–A Possible Holiday Stuffing* from Step 2, or the *Sweet Quinoa with Raisins and Toasted Almonds Stuffing* below. To complete the meal, serve it with a side of the *Cranberry Tangerine Sauce* from Step 9.

Ingredients:

1 medium-size Hokkaido pumpkin, buttercup squash, or acorn squash
Sesame or olive oil to oil the baking dish; parchment paper

Preparation:

1. Preheat oven to 350° F.
2. Cut the squash open on the top, as if making a lid, and scoop out seeds.
3. Save the top and bake it together with the rest of the squash. Cut a very thin slice off the bottom of the squash so that it sits flat.
4. Place squash in an oiled baking dish, add a small amount of water, and cover with parchment paper.
5. Bake the squash 45 minutes to 1 hour, depending on the size, until tender. Check with a fork.
6. Alternatively, cut the squash in half, scoop out seeds, and put cut side down on an oiled baking dish. Optional: season with sea salt. Add a small amount of water. Cover with parchment paper and bake at 350° F between 35–40 minutes or till tender.
7. Remove from stove and fill the squash with the sweet or savory stuffing.

Stuffing: Sweet Quinoa with Raisins and Toasted Almonds:
1 cup quinoa, thoroughly washed and rinsed (soaking optional)
2 cups filtered or spring water
Pinch sea salt
1/4 cup raisins or currants, soaked and sliced
1/2 cup toasted slivered almonds

Preparation:

• Put all in a pot except almonds, bring to a boil, and simmer for 20 minutes. Fluff quinoa with a fork, mix in the almonds, and use to stuff the pumpkin.

Steamed Rainbow-Colored Delights

4 servings

The seasonal vegetables you have in your refrigerator, like white daikon radish, parsnips, or varicolored carrots, can make this an eye-pleasing dish. Use the greens, if you can get them still attached to the roots, or add your favorite greens, like kale or collards.

Ingredients:

Filtered or spring water
Pinch sea salt
1 bunch red radishes, cleaned and sliced
1 cup leafy greens of your choice, sliced into 1½-inch pieces
2 cups carrots, julienne style
Corn kernels cut from 1 or 2 ears

Dressing:

2–4 scallions, green and white parts, sliced
2 tbsp. mellow rice or chickpea miso, mixed with 4 tbsp. cold water
1 clove garlic, pressed (optional)
1 tbsp. red wine vinegar or umeboshi vinegar
½ tbsp. tamari
1 tbsp. extra virgin olive oil

Preparation:

1. Place 2–3 inches of water in a stainless steel pot, add a pinch of sea salt, insert a vegetable steamer, and bring water to a boil.
2. Place radishes in the steamer and steam until tender but still slightly crisp.
3. Remove and set aside. Repeat this method with all the other vegetables. Steaming times may differ. (For a cold summer salad or to retain the color, drop steamed vegetables into ice water and drain.)
4. Combine all the vegetables in a serving bowl.
5. Mix the dressing ingredients with a fork and add to the vegetables. Let marinate a few minutes.
6. Serve with grain and bean dishes.

Variations:

- Combine a variety of seasonal root and green leafy vegetables.
- Use light sesame oil in the winter and raw flax oil in the summer.
- Steam some round-top vegetables like red or green cabbage.
- Add some of your favorite herbs like rosemary to the dressing.
- Choose a different dressing from Step 8 for this dish.

Breakfast or Anytime Root and Round Vegetable Dish:

Sweet-Tasting Carrot and Squash Puree

2–3 servings

This cooking style brings out the sweetness of these vegetables, giving them the ability to soothe your internal organs and energize your mind. This dish is especially good at breakfast. Let its gentle and satisfying energy carry you through the day.

Ingredients:

¼ cup onions (optional)
½ cup squash
½ cup carrots
Pinch sea salt
2 tsp. sweet rice miso, mixed with 4 tsp. cold water

Preparation:

1. Wash, scrub, and dice all the vegetables.
2. Layer onions (if using), squash, and carrots in a heavy pot.
3. Add water to half cover the vegetables, and season with a pinch of sea salt.
4. Cover the pot and bring to a boil, then lower the flame and simmer on low heat for about 20 minutes or till vegetables are soft and all liquid is absorbed.
5. Five minutes before all is ready, fold in the miso/water mix, and continue simmering until liquid is absorbed.
6. Eat vegetables as is, or mash them for a puree consistency using a hand-held blender or a suribachi.

Variations:

*   Use other seasonal vegetable combinations.
*   Oven-roast this combination for a strong winter or fall dish.

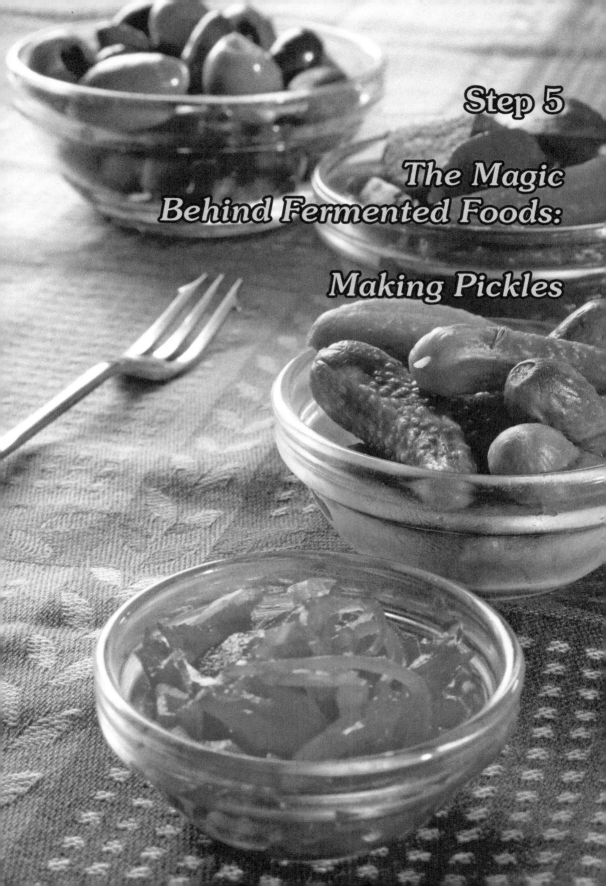

Step 5

The Magic
Behind Fermented Foods:

Making Pickles

Ah, pickles! Most people love them. You might, as we do, have fond memories of children running around with cucumber pickles in hand. Pickles are refreshing. They are also rich in probiotics and have an anti-inflammatory effect on your system. Fermenting food enhances its flavor, makes it more digestible, and is an excellent way to preserve it.

You can ferment almost anything under the sun, and there are many ways of pickling.[52] Making fermented foods in your own natural kitchen, however, needs special care, specialty tools, and careful planning. Getting organic foods is of utmost importance, as are washing the food thoroughly and using clean, sterilized cutting boards, glass containers, and well-sharpened knives. As with all food preparation, having a very clean, streamlined kitchen makes your home fires strong. During this Step, we concentrate on how to make quick short-time pickles. They are easily made in your kitchen and good to eat year-round. You can also purchase many pickled and fermented foods. Look for good quality products that are unpasteurized, traditionally made, and free of sugar, chemicals, and preservatives.

Store them in a cool room, pantry, or refrigerator, and use them to garnish and complement your meals. One (or two) tablespoon of fermented pickles with your meal is a sufficient serving for most adults. Depending on the age of the children, they need low- or no-salt pickles, in smaller amounts.

Histories and Names of Some Fermented Foods

The various processes of pickling and fermenting food were developed, often by chance, before refrigeration and transportation of foods was the norm. A wide range of foods, including fruits, fish, dairy, meats, grains, and beans, are still being pickled and fermented by almost all cultures around the world.

Familiar fermented foods include sauerkraut, pickled ginger, *kvass, kefir, kombucha,* yogurt, buttermilk, sourdough bread, *tempeh*, miso, tamari, soy sauce, *natto*, olives, chocolate, coffee, tea, and even *togwa,* a fermented gruel from Tanzania. On and on goes the list of the fermented foods that have long-standing traditions.

Archives 10,000 years old affirm that vinegar is one of the oldest fermented foods, right after wine or mead. The health benefits of vinegar are numerous, but be sure to look for traditionally and naturally produced vinegars that often still contain the "mother culture."

Records show that Romans ate sauerkraut, and that it was a staple in medieval Europe. Genghis Khan is said to have used it around 1200 AD, and it helped prevent scurvy on the long sea excursions of Captain John Cook during the eighteenth century.

In China, cabbage has been fermented for thousands of years. *Kimchi*, a traditional fermented Korean dish that is still eaten in small amounts with many meals, is also used in other Asian countries, and has become a favorite in the West as well. It is generally made with Napa (Chinese) cabbage, but can contain a variety of other vegetables such as radishes, scallions, or cucumbers. Spices are added for flavor and additional preservation. One of the oldest references to kimchi dates to 1000 BC.

The Magic behind Fermented Pickles!

The magic behind making fermented pickles is sea salt plus time and/or pressure. This combination promotes the growth of important bacteria like *lactobacilli,* which ferment the food, and it helps to develop health-promoting enzymes. You get the best results with this method when food is pickled for three to four days. The process also makes raw food more digestible and enhances its flavor. To alter the sour taste of pickles, add a variety of flavors such as salty, sweet, sweet and sour, spicy, bitter, and pungent.

Vinegars are made from various fermented fruits and vegetables, and contain *acetic acid.* Vinegars, with their distinct sour taste, are used as pickling agents to preserve and add flavor to vegetables and other foods. Vinegars are also used as a condiment, in dressings, or in medicinal tonics. Some, such as apple cider vinegar and umeboshi vinegar, aid digestion and have a cleansing effect on the body, if they are not pasteurized and still contain the mother of vinegar bacterial culture. Be cautious about overusing them, however, as their acid content can be damaging to skin and internal organs.

Fermenting food is a great way to store harvest surplus, and provides variety in preserved foods in combination with canning, drying, or freezing. It also may preserve some nutrients, such as vitamin C that is destroyed by heat, more than other home food preservation methods.

Fermented Foods for Health-Conscious Eating

In today's era of health-conscious eating, the fermented *kombucha* beverage that originated in Japan and North China, made with mutually beneficial cultures of bacteria and yeast, is a sought-after drink to improve digestion. Varieties of the fermented grain drink *rejuvelac,* originally from Europe, are also beneficial. Rejuvelac can be made with millet, buckwheat, rice, quinoa, or gluten-containing grains like barley and rye. A sweet, thick, creamy fermented rice beverage called *amazake* (Japanese for "sweet sake") is very popular in macrobiotic and natural foods cooking. Use amazake as a natural sweetener for pies, puddings (see Step 9 for recipe), and other dishes, or just drink it, cool or warmed. These drinks can also be used as starters to make other fermented foods. They have a more yin quality than the fermented foods like miso or tamari described below. Use them according to the season, your condition, and your liking.

Traditional Japanese fermented foods that have a more yang character are miso, tamari, soy sauce, umeboshi plums, umeboshi vinegar, white daikon radish pickle (*takuan*), tempeh, and natto. These should all have a regular place in your macrobiotic natural foods kitchen. Add them to a variety of soups, grains, beans, and vegetable dishes to enhance flavor and digestibility.

Miso, a fermented bean or grain paste, which is mostly known for its use in *miso soup,* is available in a variety of flavors and fermentation times. Buy traditionally made, naturally fermented, unpasteurized, nonhomogenized miso varieties that are made with organic beans, grains, and sea salt and a fermentation agent called *koji.* You can use miso in all seasons and for all reasons. The most health-promoting miso is fermented a long time, between two to three years, like the brown rice (*genmai*), barley (*mugi*) (contains gluten), and soybean (*hatcho*) miso. They have a strong, salty taste (yang) and are good to eat regularly, especially during the colder months.

During warm weather, good choices for soups, sauces, and dips are short-time fermented, sweeter-tasting (yin) light or mellow rice miso or chickpea miso. These are fermented for three to six months and contain less salt. For variety, mix a long-time fermented miso with a short-time fermented miso.

Tamari, traditionally a byproduct of miso production, is another fermented seasoning agent to use daily or often in soups, or to flavor other dishes. Tamari provides a tasty and healthy gluten-free alternative to fermented soy sauce and shoyu, which contain wheat. The recipes in this book call for tamari in recognition of the gluten-conscious aspect of this book. However, if your health permits it, you can use soy sauce or shoyu instead. *Nama* brand soy sauce (contains gluten) is a raw, fermented soy and wheat product that is great to use for raw food preparation methods. If you are gluten and soy intolerant, try coconut sauce that has a similar taste and texture.

Umeboshi plum, a fruit related to the apricot, is pickled from six months to two years with sea salt after drying for three or four days. The umeboshi plum enhances the flavor and digestibility of foods. Umeboshi byproducts are the salty and sour *umeboshi vinegar* and the crushed *umeboshi paste*. All three forms are health-supportive fermented foods to use in your kitchen as seasonings, condiments, home remedies, or as pickling agents.

Sauerkraut, sourdough bread, and beer—even pickled herring—are well-known fermented foods associated with German cuisine. Add sauerkraut, raw or cooked, to your meals often.

Gluten Advice: Soy sauce and shoyu contain gluten. If this is a concern, use tamari, which is a gluten-free soy sauce. The recipes in this book contain tamari. Barley miso also contains gluten—use brown rice miso, hatcho miso, adzuki bean miso, or chickpea miso instead. Most sourdough breads and beer contain gluten.

Health Aspects of Fermented and Pickled Foods

Pros:

- Raw, fermented foods are rich in enzymes and antioxidants and strengthen the immune system. They help to remove toxins from food and from your body and provide anti-aging benefits.
- A few tablespoons of raw pickled foods per meal or per day will stimulate your digestive juices to flow. As these foods help to restore proper bacterial balance in your gut, they improve your digestive process and the absorption of food. If you have proper intestinal flora, then B vitamins such as folic acid, riboflavin, niacin, and biotin are assimilated more easily.
- Fermenting by soaking whole grains, beans, and legumes neutralizes their phytic acid content and makes them more digestible. This process helps to release powerful nutrients and ensure the absorption of zinc, calcium, iron, and magnesium. Soak, ferment, and cook beans and grains together, as they build a complete protein with all the essential amino acids for human nutrition. See Steps 2 and 3 for further information on soaking, and recipes.

Cons:

- Pickled food tastes so good that it's easy to eat too much. Pickles are made with a salt-containing agent, and eating a large amount can make you feel contracted and throw you off balance. Capers, olives, and umeboshi plums can be very high in salt. If you are on a low-salt diet, keep these foods to a minimum, or soak them or rinse them in water to minimize their saltiness.
- Use caution if you have candida or other digestive issues, as you might be sensitive to fermented foods, which can contain yeasts and mold.
- Children should eat only pickles that are low in salt or are soaked in water. They should eat less than a teaspoon of pickles at one time. Don't give pickles to children under the age of three.

Embrace Culinary Traditions As a Way of Life

Fermented and pickled foods are often one of the easiest avenues for incorporating foods from cultures around the globe. Just think about coffee, tea, chocolate, and wine, which are all fermented foods. When you embrace another culture's culinary tradition at the same time you cultivate your own, you can harmonize with the foods of other civilizations and live more peacefully on this earth. Michio Kushi says, "If we are open to that idea, we can embrace in that way all the traditions of this earth, and thus we can also harmonize and live in peace on this earth."[53]

The Yin and Yang of Raw, Fermented, and Cooked Foods

Raw foods provide more enzymes and vitamins than foods cooked with high heat (over 115° F). You will notice, though, that if you do choose to eat mostly raw foods in all seasons, it is often difficult to achieve balance. According to the macrobiotic principles of yin and yang, raw foods have yin energy and are energetically balancing during the hot, yang summer seasons. In colder weather you naturally want to eat cooked foods, whereas during hot summers eating some raw, cold foods seems more appealing. Paying attention to this dynamic will provide more balance. Fermenting raw foods by making pickles, with salt and adding pressure and time makes them more digestible and adding more yang energy and thus easier to eat in all seasons.

Balance Is the Key Word

When you are eating too many raw uncooked foods (yin) and your constitution or condition is too yin, you will not be able to produce enough warmth (yang energy), and your health might suffer. A yin condition can easily occur when eating too many fruits and raw foods in cold weather, but really at any time of the year, even summer.

If you are used to a heavy meat-centered way of life (yang), and your condition is very yang, you might be able to handle more raw, yin foods for a while, until your condition is fairly balanced. Raw foods (yin) can increase the discharge of toxins from animal foods (yang).

A *raw food cleanse* can be done using raw juices or raw dishes as a specific treatment for certain ailments. If you would like to experiment with a raw food cleanse, do it under supervision and not for a long time; a safe maximum for most people would be three to six days. Judge the results for yourself. A raw foods cleanse is best done during the warmer or hotter season. After your cleanse, you can slowly start using a variety of cooking methods for seasonal foods with different applications of heat.

Every day, eat a couple of spoonfuls or a few pieces of fermented and pickled raw foods to provide easy-to-digest enzymes and fresh vitamins. Enhance your cooked food with fresh raw garnishes, herbs, edible flower decorations, or dressings using parsley, scallions, basil, chives, or finely sliced or grated raw daikon or other vegetables.

Cooking with Fermented Foods

Be very careful when you heat fermented foods. Using high heat, around 115–145° F, especially for a long time, destroys the enzymes and affects the taste. So choose uncooked and live fermented foods often to receive their full benefits. If you use a fermented product in your cooked and hot dishes, always add it toward the end of cooking and a minute after the food has stopped boiling. Cook on low heat or simmer for only a short time. (If you would like to add the fermented product for just its taste, cooking it longer is fine.)

The world-famous miso soup is a great way to have a warm fermented beverage. See recipe below, and more miso soup ideas are in Step 7. Many recipes in this book are also flavored with a variety of miso or tamari. A great warm fermented dish that blends East and West cuisines is *Arame Sea Vegetable with Tempeh and Sauerkraut* (recipe in Step 6). When you cook with miso, sauerkraut, or other fermented foods, add them toward the end of cooking, and keep the heat on low for just a short time to preserve enzymes and taste. You can enjoy miso and sauerkraut for both taste and nutrition.

Seasonal Reflections on
What Kind Of Pickles to Eat and When

Because you can pickle almost anything, you will never run out of scrumptious possibilities. Choose the vegetables and other foods you like and pickle them in your kitchen according to the current season. Since there is a wide variety of food available during the warmer months, you can make one- to two-week refrigerator pickles then. Short-term pickled, fermented, marinated, pressed raw salads are also very supportive for a balanced system. They can add an uplifting feeling during any season of the year.

Great to eat all year round, but especially in the winter months, are long-time fermented foods like sauerkraut, daikon radish takuan pickles, and umeboshi plums. These pickled foods are important parts of a nourishing diet. You can buy them in natural food stores or online, or make them at home. You can pickle root vegetables like carrots or daikon radish in miso for three months or longer. Use more yang miso like soy miso, barley miso (contains gluten) or dark red rice miso, fermented between two or three years, or over two summers, most often in the colder months. For lighter fare or during the hotter season or in-between seasons like late summer, try short-time fermented, unpasteurized miso such as sweet rice or chickpea in your soups or for fermenting vegetables. Make brine pickles with water and salt in warmer months. Reserve herbed, garlic, or spiced pickles for special occasions only, or eat now and then during the hot summer.

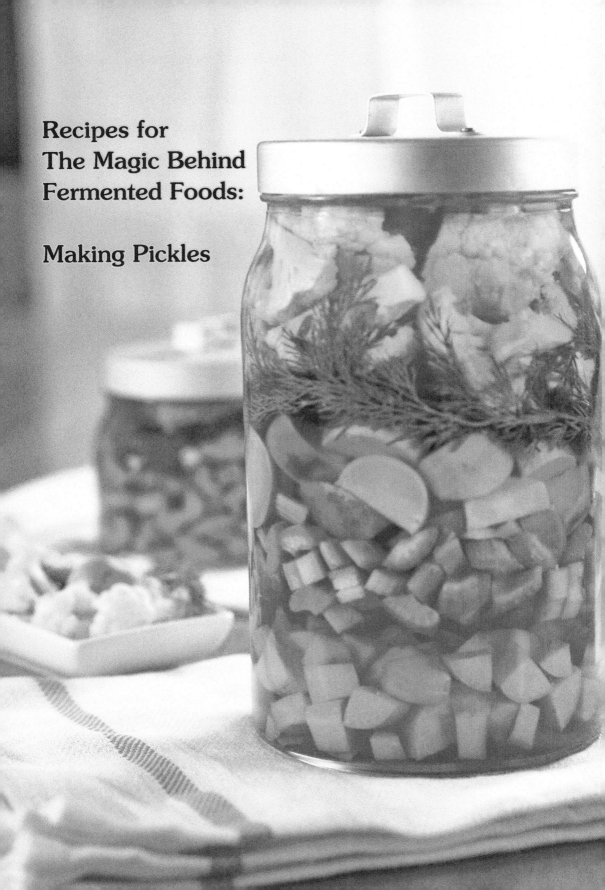

Recipes for
The Magic Behind
Fermented Foods:

Making Pickles

Refrigerator Pickles – Seasonal Vegetables in Umeboshi Plum Brine (Photo p. 103)

Suggested serving: 1 tablespoon with meals

Umeboshi plum vinegar, made from plums that are long-time fermented, up to 2 years, is an excellent base for these pickles. Eating umeboshi plums regularly can restore your digestive health, help to prevent nausea, and provide relief from systemic toxicity.

Ingredients:

2 cups filtered or spring water
5 tbsp. umeboshi plum vinegar
½ tsp. sea salt (optional)
½ cup carrots, diced
½ cup celery, diced
½ cup red radishes, diced
2 cups cauliflower, cut into small florets
Dill, several sprigs
Quart-size Mason jar with lid and cheesecloth

Preparation:

1. Boil water. Cool to room temperature and add the umeboshi vinegar and optional sea salt.
2. Layer carrots, celery, radishes, sprig of dill, and cauliflower in a Mason jar and add the water-vinegar mixture.
3. Cover the jar with cheesecloth and close with the lid rim. Place in a cool place or refrigerate.
4. After one day, check the taste, and if needed, adjust plum vinegar according to your preference.
5. Remove cheesecloth, close with the lid, and place in a cool place or refrigerate.
6. In 3–7 days, or after vegetables have lost their rawness but are still crunchy, they are ready.
7. If vegetables taste too salty and strong, rinse or place in fresh water before serving.

Variations:

- Instead of umeboshi vinegar, use rice vinegar, red wine vinegar, apple cider vinegar, or soak 6–8 umeboshi plums in hot water for two hours before adding vegetables.
- Add onions, cucumber, corn, or other seasonal vegetables.
- Add parsley, chives, and black peppercorns, ginger, or red chili pepper.

Raw Pickled Burdock Root

4 side servings

Burdock is a wild plant native to Europe and Northern Asia. It grows as a weed, but cultivated roots are available in stores and eaten in vegetable dishes. Burdock root (Japanese **gobo**) is also frequently used in concoctions as a detoxifier or blood purifier and even added to poultices.

Ingredients:

1 burdock root
2 tbsp. or more rice vinegar
1/3 cup white onions or shallots
Garnish: green parts of scallion, finely sliced
Garnish: toasted sesame seeds

Preparation:

1. Scrub the dark brown burdock root vigorously with a vegetable brush under water to remove dirt and some of the skin. To completely remove skin, use a vegetable peeler.

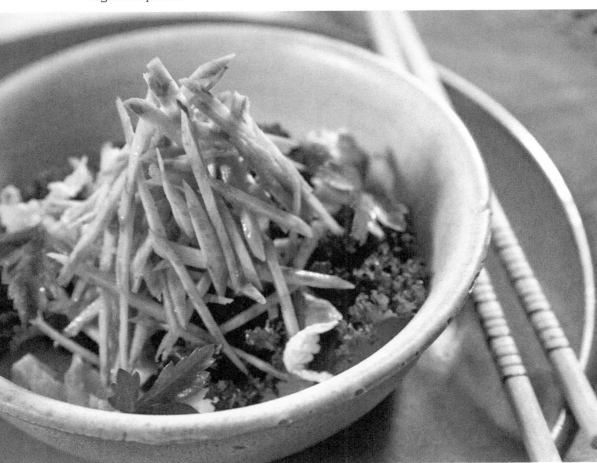

2. Trim both ends and slice into very fine julienne-style (matchstick) pieces.
3. As you work, drop burdock immediately into a bowl of rice vinegar to prevent discoloration and oxidation. The rice vinegar will also help to ferment the burdock.
4. Add finely sliced raw white onions or shallots.
5. Pickle for 1–7 days.
6. To serve, remove vegetables and garnish with freshly sliced scallion greens and a sprinkle of toasted sesame seeds.

Variations:

• Pickle the burdock with umeboshi vinegar for a slight pink color, or use lemon juice.
• Try this pickling method with other seasonal root vegetables from Step 4.

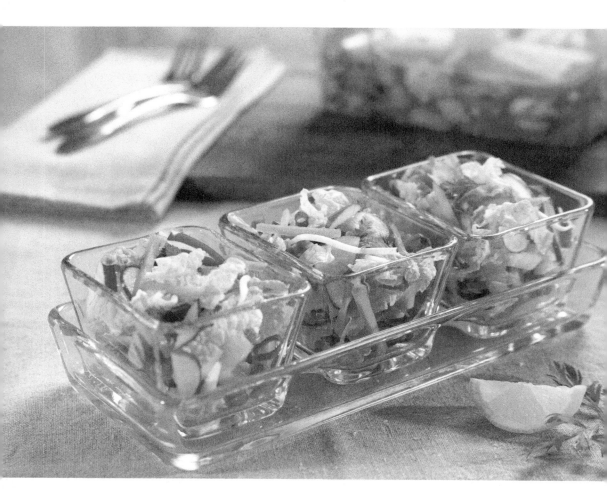

Lemony Marinated Cabbage Salad with Julienne Carrots

8 side servings

Serve this raw fermented salad year round as a small side dish. It can also provide a refreshing snack in the afternoon. For a coleslaw effect, add *Dairy and Egg-Free Vegan Mayonnaise* from Step 8, p. 162.

Ingredients:
2 cups Napa (Chinese) cabbage
½ cup carrots, julienne style
½ cup red radishes, sliced
3 scallions, both the green and white parts, finely sliced
½ tsp. sea salt, or to taste
Juice of one lemon, or to taste; zest of one lemon (optional)
1 tbsp. tamari, or to taste (optional)
1 tsp. dulse sea vegetable flakes (optional)

Preparation:
1. Wash and slice cabbage into 1-inch slices, then towel dry or spin in a salad spinner.
2. Place julienne-cut carrots, radishes, cabbage, and scallions into a mixing bowl.
3. Add sea salt and lemon juice, lemon zest, tamari, and dulse flakes, if using, and mix and press gently with your hands.
4. Use a salad press, or press vegetables with a plate with a heavy weight on top. Press for about 1 hour before serving, or until some water is expelled, but dish is still crunchy. If too salty, rinse the vegetables.
5. Keeps in the refrigerator for one week. With continued pressing and fermentation, the crunchiness will be minimized.

Variations:
- Use vinegar—umeboshi, rice, or apple cider—as an alternative to lemon juice.
- Use finely sliced green or red cabbage instead of Napa cabbage.
- Try fermenting seasonal combinations of vegetables like celery, carrots, or cauliflower.

Sea Salt-Pressed Red Radishes

4 side servings

Red radishes with their deep red color provide a tasty and beautiful visual on your plate.

Ingredients:
2 cups red radishes, sliced
Green tops of the radishes or equal amount of kale, finely sliced
1 tsp. sea salt
Sprinkles of dulse sea vegetable flakes (optional)
Garnish: scallions, sliced

Preparation:

1. Put radishes and greens into a large bowl and mix and press with hands, adding the sea salt and, if using, dulse flakes.
2. Fit a plate with a heavy weight on top of the vegetables to press them, or use a salad press.
3. Press to marinate for at least one hour before serving. If too salty, rinse before serving.
4. Keeps in the refrigerator for one week. Serve as a side dish with sliced scallions.

Variations:

- Use white daikon radish with umeboshi vinegar instead of sea salt for an eye-pleasing pink color.
- Instead of sea salt, use adjusted amounts of umeboshi vinegar, plums, or paste; tamari; lemon juice or rind; or other vinegar.
- Press other roots like carrots or turnips, or rounds like onions, or green leafy vegetables.

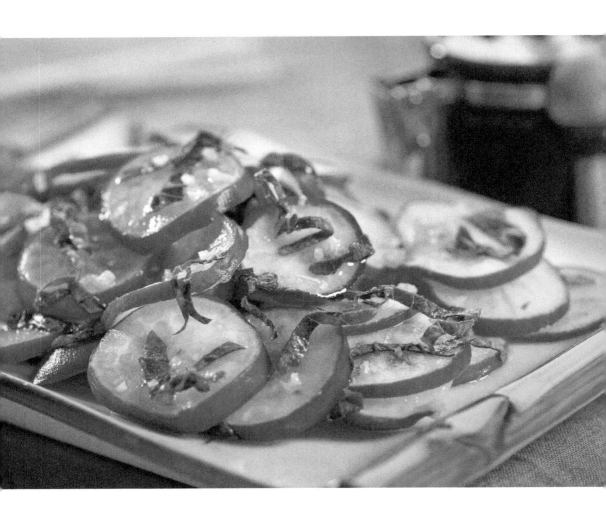

Homemade Fermented Tofu Cheese on Cucumber Slices

4 side servings

This is the best vegan cheese and has the added benefits of the fermented miso. It is a healthy choice, preferred over the chemically processed tofu cheeses available in the markets. It can be a base for a variety of other dishes. By mashing in olives or basil, for instance, you can also serve it as a dip for crackers or vegetables.

Ingredients:
1 cake fresh hard tofu (1 lb.)
2 cups chickpea miso or dark miso
1 large English cucumber
Garnish: long pieces of chives

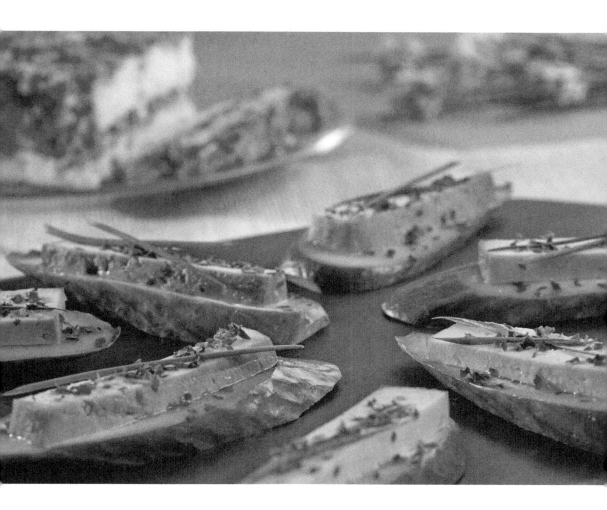

Preparation:

1. Rinse tofu and place between two plates or cutting boards and press with the weight of a heavy object for at least 30 minutes, then towel dry.
2. Apply miso around all sides of the tofu cake and store covered in a cool place 2–3 days, depending on your desired taste.
3. Remove the miso and save for further use.
4. Cut the tofu cake into ¼-inch slices (about 8 slices per cake) and then cut into quarters.
5. Cut the cucumber into slices on the diagonal, ¼ inch thick.
6. Place a quarter-size piece of tofu cheese on a slice of raw cucumber.
7. Cut a few 4-inch pieces of chives as garnish.
8. As hors d'oeuvres, serve 4 pieces per person.

Variations:

- Use different kinds of miso according to taste preference. Hatcho (soy bean) miso has the strongest quality, and chickpea miso is the lightest.
- Instead of an English cucumber, use a slicing cucumber.

Fermented Recipes for Breakfast or Anytime Dishes!

Quickest Cup of Miso Soup

1 serving

Heat one cup of water. Add 1 tsp. of miso of your choice and sprinkles of wakame flakes. Add finely cubed soft tofu. Add (optional) watercress or finely shredded Napa (Chinese) cabbage. These greens are easy to clean and require minimum cooking time, yet add a great contrast and further nutrients.

Soft Cooked Grain with Umeboshi Plum

2 servings

Any whole grain prepared as soft grain porridge with the added benefits of umeboshi is great dish for breakfast, and especially if you are not feeling well.

Ingredients:

1 cup cooked whole grain
2 cups filtered or spring water
4 tsp. umeboshi paste or mashed umeboshi plum, to taste
Garnish: sliced scallions; nori sea vegetable cut into small strips (optional)

Preparation:
1. Bring the water and grain to a boil, and then simmer for 20 minutes or until soft. Then return heat to low setting.
2. Mash umeboshi plum with a little warm water and add to grain.
3. Mix, and simmer on very low heat for 5 minutes. The porridge should not taste salty.
4. Before serving, add scallions and, if using, nori strips for garnish.

Variations:
- Add a variety of finely chopped seasonal vegetables and cook as above.
- Add a small amount of miso to the mix instead of the umeboshi plum.

Rice Miso-Infused Tahini Sesame Paté
4 side servings

Use this protein-rich paté served on toast or as a dip with vegetables like carrots or celery for a different kind of breakfast. Serve it with crackers, apple slices, or chips as a snack or a hors d'oeuvre.

Ingredients:
3 tbsp. tahini sesame paste, raw (or roasted)
2 tbsp., or to taste, light rice miso or miso flavor of your choice
2 tbsp. filtered or spring water; adjust amount if needed
Garnish: scallions or parsley, minced

Preparation:
1. Mix all ingredients in suribachi or food processor.
2. Add water, miso, and tahini to reach the preferred consistency and taste.
3. Serve with toast, wraps, or rice cakes, and garnish with minced scallions or parsley.

Variations:
- Grate and squeeze ginger juice for a light, spicy flavor, or lemon juice for a citrus flavor.
- Add grated apples right before serving for a hint of sweetness.

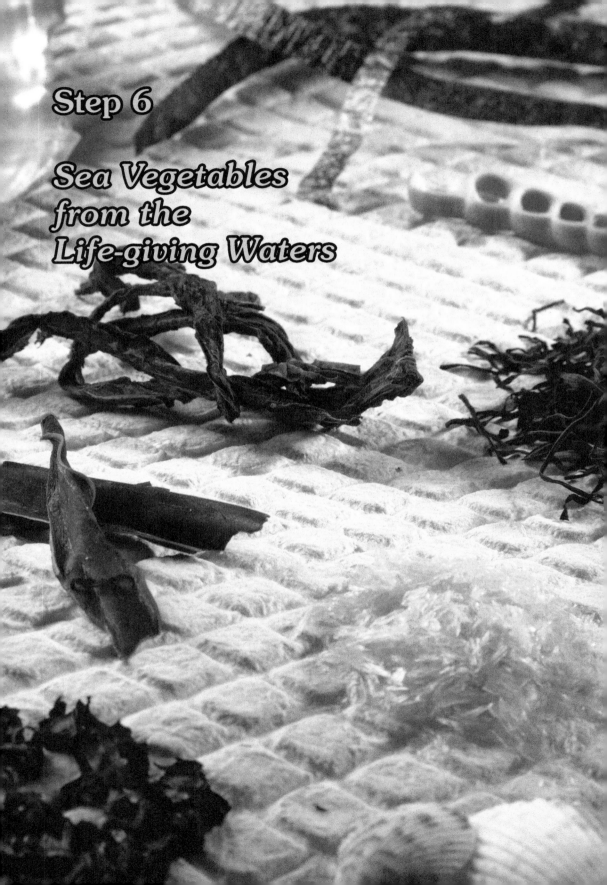

Step 6

Sea Vegetables from the Life-giving Waters

Plants from the sea could be the most foreign food you eat, depending on where you live. Although many people value sea vegetables, nibbling on seaweed might not be the picture you have in mind when thinking about a healthy lifestyle. In many Asian families, however, sea vegetables are eaten like green beans and carrots in the West. If you like sushi, you have probably eaten nori, the sea vegetable that wraps around maki sushi.

Sea vegetables can have a profound positive impact on your nourishment and well-being with their amino acids, enzymes, and minerals like calcium, magnesium, iron, iodine, potassium, and zinc, as well as vitamins A, B, E, and K. They also contain a complete spectrum of trace minerals that are inconsistently available in land vegetables. You can receive their protective power as they help you to fulfill your mineral and other nutritional needs by eating about one tablespoon of dried sea vegetables per adult per meal every day.

Throughout this book, many of the recipes call for adding small amounts of sea vegetables, especially kombu, for flavor, nutrient enhancement, and digestibility. In many cases, the only one who will know about these "extra" ingredients is you, the cook. Specifically during this Step, familiarize yourself with other ways to prepare sea vegetables in your kitchen. Experiment by using them as a side dish as you would with land vegetables, and to make snacks and condiments.

History of Sea Vegetables

Sea vegetables have been valued in many traditions for thousands of years as a source of minerals and for their ability to enrich and cleanse the blood. Archaeological findings suggest that Japanese cultures have been eating them for more than 10,000 years. But this food is not limited to Asia. Coastal dwellers all over the world—in Chile, Hawaii, and New Zealand; North America; and northern Europe in France, Ireland, Scotland, Norway, and Iceland—have been harvesting sea vegetables since ancient times.[54] Sea vegetables have had other uses too, such as medicines and fertilizers, and were traded far inland. There are historical accounts of North American Indians, Celts, Vikings, Hawaiian kings, Chinese royalty, and Irish monks, all savoring and trading these native foods.[55] [56] [57] [58]

Names of Edible Sea Plants and Where to Get Them

Vegetables from the sea—sea plants, sea vegetables, also called seaweed—grow in all oceans and seas, from the equator to the Arctic. Some varieties are also found in freshwater lakes. They can grow in shallow water or on the ocean floor as long as the sunlight can penetrate; like all plants, they need light to live.

They belong to a diverse group of ancient water plants known as algae. There are thousands of types of algae, and the sea vegetables are classified into categories by color: brown, red, or green. It is helpful to know the different names for the same or similar types of sea vegetables when shopping for them. For instance, *kombu* is kelp, *wakame* is alaria, and *nori* is laver. In the recipes we use the Japanese names.

Familiarize yourself with the most popular edible types during this Step: *arame* (lacy, wiry strands), *hijiki* (thicker, black strands), *kombu* or *kelp* (dark, hard strips), *wakame* or *alaria* (soft strips or flakes), *mekabu* (wakame flowering sprout), *dulse* (red sheets or flakes), *nori* or *laver* (dark purple-black flat sheet that turns iridescent green when toasted), *agar-agar* (flakes or pressed into translucent bars), *sea palm* (dark flat strands), and *sea lettuce* (light green leaves).

Get these sea vegetables from natural food stores or reputable online sources. Buy from companies that harvest sustainably, preferably in ecologically protected seas where development is forbidden, to ensure future generations of edible seaweed sourcing. From many shores throughout the world you can find socially responsible farming companies providing clean, highly edible sea vegetables.

Look for organic certification on the package as an indication of monitoring for possible herbicide, pesticide, heavy metal, radioactive components, and bacteriological contamination in harvesting and handling wild sea vegetables.[59] As sea vegetables are sold mostly dried, they have a long shelf life and are also good survival foods. Store them in tightly sealed glass containers or plastic bags, out of direct light and moisture, to retain their freshness.

Seaweed companies also harvest and prepare these plants for fodder, fertilizers, cosmetics, and a variety of other industrial uses. Seaweed extracts like agar, alginate, and carrageenan are used widely in food and pharmaceutical products.[60]

Nutrient Content and Health Benefits of the Most Popular Sea Vegetables

Sea vegetables, usually eaten in small portions, can be a major source of minerals and some other nutrients in the daily diet. Most sea veggies, especially nori, are excellent for vegans, as they provide up to ten times more calcium and iron by weight than milk.

Nori/Laver. A good source of calcium, iron, potassium, and iodine; high in vitamins B, C, and D; with more vitamin A than carrots; richer in protein than soybeans, milk, meat, fish, or poultry. All sea vegetables have significant amounts (1–3%) of omega-3 and omega-6 fatty acids. Nori, in particular, has 3% omega-3 fatty acids.

Kombu/Kelp. Contains vitamins A, D, C, K, and B; is a good source of the trace elements copper, zinc, and chromium; and is high in calcium, iron, and all major minerals. It can assist with blood pressure regulation, digestion and colon cleansing, and weight loss.

Dulse. Good source of vitamins E, C, A and B-complex; extremely high in vitamin B6; as well as potassium, fluoride, magnesium, calcium, dietary fiber, and protein. It is a superior source of iron and iodine. Unlike other seaweeds, it is relatively low in sodium. Iodine is essential for thyroid gland health and thyroid hormone secretion. It strengthens the blood, adrenals, and kidneys, and provides help in treating herpes and temporary relief of gum or tooth pain if put directly on the area.

Wakame/Alaria. Is low in saturated fat and very low in cholesterol, but very high in sodium. It is also a good source of vitamins A, C, and K; B vitamins; vitamin E (alpha tocopherol); niacin, pantothenic acid, and phosphorus; and a very good source of riboflavin, folate, calcium, iron, magnesium, copper, and manganese. Wakame is said to be a "woman's seaweed."

Agar-agar. Is low in sodium, and very low in saturated fat and cholesterol. It is also a good source of vitamin E (alpha tocopherol), vitamin K, pantothenic acid, zinc, and copper, and a very good source of folate, calcium, iron, magnesium, potassium, and manganese. Helps to strengthen bones.

Arame. Arame is low in sodium and carbohydrate, and fat free. It is rich in dietary fiber, and a good source of vitamin A, magnesium, and calcium. It is also a source of potassium, iron, iodine, vitamin B2, mannitol (noncaloric sugar alcohol), zinc, and many trace minerals. It contains the polysaccharide laminarin and the tripeptide eisenin. It is rich in lignans, which help fight cancer. This mineral-rich vegetable is traditionally used to help relieve kidney and bladder-related disorders.

Hijiki. Has one of the highest concentrations of calcium and iron of any food and is an excellent source of minerals and trace elements, as well as vitamins A, C, and B. It helps reduce serum cholesterol and prevent heart disease.

Research on Sea Vegetables

Pros:

- **Iodine.** Sea vegetables are the richest plant source of iodine in the world. Iodine is an essential mineral for life, and having the right amount of iodine in your body is important to support the immune system and thyroid function. It is needed in every cell to prevent cancer. Low iodine, like low zinc, is associated with lower intelligence and behavior problems, depression, fatigue, and many other serious conditions. The right amount of iodine in your body can also protect you against radioactive contamination. People often don't have enough iodine, but iodine supplementation or enrichment is not as natural a source of iodine as sea vegetables. Iodine-rich sea vegetables have been used to treat goiter (iodine deficiency) in inland China for centuries. China has many kelp seaweed farms. Kelp/kombu is particularly high in iodine and is considered the best natural source of iodine in the world, as it contains around 2500 mcg/gm.

- **Trace minerals.** When you eat unprocessed dried sea vegetables, you can benefit from their many healing properties and profound positive impact on your nourishment with their complete spectrum of trace minerals not available in land vegetables. They are highly valued around the world. Dr. Weston Price, who is known for his dietary research in unique places and populations, found that natives from the high Andes consumed small quantities of sea vegetables every day. With much difficulty, they obtained this seaweed from their coastal neighbors and carried it in small bags around their necks.[61]

- **Immune system.** Sea vegetables can boost an immune system function that is impaired due to inadequate minerals either in the diet or in the body.

- **Cleanser.** The high levels of alginic acid found in seaweed are known to act as an intestinal cleanser. They can help the body to eliminate accumulated toxins, as they bind heavy metals such as cadmium and radioactive pollutants like strontium that are present in the environment from industry and transport them from the body. Sea vegetables also contain cleansing phytonutrients and fat-metabolizing and fat-eliminating polysaccharides like fucoidan that work in combination with the trace minerals.[62 63 64 65]

- The **naturally occurring flavor enhancer** in kombu, an unbound glutamic acid, can also be found in Parmesan cheese, peas, tomatoes, grapes, and plums. Small amounts of this naturally occurring glutamic acid in kombu have not been shown to be harmful to the body. In contrast, research shows that larger quantities of the synthetic, manufactured monosodium glutamate (MSG) that is often added to enhance the flavor of foods in restaurants as well as in mass-produced food products has unfavorable effects on nerve cell development, both alone and synergistically in combination with other food additives.[66]

- **Anticancer effects.** Japanese scientists reported that several varieties of kombu and mojaban, common sea vegetables eaten in Asia and traditionally used in a decoction for cancer in Chinese herbal medicine, were effective in the treatment of tumors in laboratory experiments.[67] Dr. Jane Teas of Harvard University suggested that kelp (kombu) and wakame consumption might be a factor in the lower rates of breast cancer in Japan. Sea vegetables are very high in lignans, plant substances that become phytoestrogens in the body, meaning they help to block the chemical estrogens that can predispose people to cancers such as breast cancer.[68]

Cons:

- **Sodium.** Because it comes from the sea, seaweed contains sodium. Consumption should be minimized by anyone on a sodium-restricted diet. Wakame has the highest sodium content, with kombu (kelp) and nori (laver) having significantly less.
- **Iodine.** In a small number of susceptible individuals, excess dietary iodine may result in reversible hypothyroidism.[69]
- **B12.** Sea vegetables are sometimes mentioned as a source of vitamin B12, but there are conflicting studies about its bioavailability to humans. It is probably not a reliable source of this vitamin.[70][71] If you are on a vegan diet, please check your levels and consult a professional to find appropriate supplementation if needed.

Sea Vegetable Way of Life Inspirations

- Spend time often by a river, sea, lake, or ocean.
- Vacation by the sea, or search for a place where you can attend a sea vegetable harvest.
- Seek out natural sea vegetable cosmetics like kelp conditioner, shampoo, soaps and facial scrubs, and lotions and creams. Indulge in a Sea Vegetable Therapy Bath (see recipe in Step 10)
- Use seaweed in your pet's food and notice amazing results on its health and well-being.
- Use seaweed as fertilizer in your garden. It works best in loose, sandy soils. The magnetic energy of seaweed connects with the soil, and its many trace minerals provide healthy foods for your table.

Portions and Other Aspects of Cooking Sea Vegetables

Eat nori, wakame, kombu, and dulse sea vegetables regularly or daily to accent your beans, soups, vegetable dishes, or as condiments or snacks. Make arame, hijiki, and agar-agar sea vegetable dishes occasionally. Sea vegetables provide enhancement to flavor and nutrients, and they are easy to "sneak into" your dishes.

Nori. Eat ½-1 sheet of nori—daily. Nori is made from seaweed that is pressed into sheets and then air-dried in the sun at low temperatures and with enzymes intact. It is best to toast it before eating. Sheets usually come in raw form, so you will probably need to brush it over a gas flame or a heated electric plate for a few moments until it turns from black to green. You can nibble or snack on nori just like that—a sheet will provide you with minerals and great energy. Eat instead of chips, and give them to your kids. Shred a sheet and sprinkle over grains or soups, or buy nori flakes or powder. Make a Soft Nori Condiment to eat with your grain dishes, or make a Sea Vegetable Roll. (See the recipes in this Step.)

Wakame. *Add 1 teaspoon of wakame to soups or salads—daily.* Wakame is a milder-tasting relative of kombu, and both are native to the Far East. It has a soft leafy structure with a strong center. A similar plant, alaria, grows in the Atlantic Ocean. Wakame is sold in longer dried strips that need to be soaked in cold water for three minutes and sliced. It is also available in convenient instant flakes. It tastes delicious and is easy to add to soups, salads, land vegetables, or prepared as a condiment. Like kombu, it can tenderize a bean dish. It can be used as a mineral-rich (with a lower iodine content) table condiment by baking it in the oven and then crushing it into a powder. Sprinkle it over grain dishes. Use mekabu, the root of wakame, occasionally in your dishes and for strengthening your nervous system.

Kombu. *Add a stamp-size piece of kombu to beans, soups, or vegetable dishes—daily.* Kombu, known for its famed *umami* taste, or "fifth flavor," is a naturally occurring flavor enhancer that comes in thick, dark green strips. Cut it into your preferred shape, give it a quick rinse or wipe, and/or a 10-minute soaking, depending on the recipe. It cooks in about 30–40 minutes. It is well known that adding a small strip of kombu to beans will enhance their flavor, help soften them, and make them more digestible. Plus, its extremely rich mineral content brings balance to the high protein of legumes. Prepare condiments by baking the dried kombu and grinding it into a powder, or cooking it finely sliced with tamari and ginger, as in *Shio Kombu*. Deep-fry it and serve it as a crispy snack, or prepare a *kombu dashi* for a soup stock.

Dulse. *Sprinkle as a condiment on grain dishes or add to salad dressings and greens—occasionally.* Dulse is a red sea vegetable that grows wild along the middle to lower shores in many parts of Europe such as Ireland, Scotland, and Iceland, and on the North Atlantic coasts of Canada and New England.[72] You can get it as whole leaves to eat as is, or toast it and eat as a crispy snack or in soups. It also comes in convenient flakes, to sprinkle on whole grains, pasta, salads, vegetables, and even popcorn.

Arame. *Use arame to make a one-third cup side dish—two to three times per week.* Arame is a mineral-rich brown sea vegetable that is washed, dried naturally in air and sun, and then steamed for five hours to soften it and enhance its color. It makes its way to our markets in finely shredded form. This makes it easy to use. A quick rinse or light soaking is all it needs to rehydrate for cooking with seasonal vegetables. In the summer, you can wash and soak it and eat it as a raw salad with vegetables and a dressing.

Hijiki. *Use in a small side dish—every 5-10 days.* As hijiki has a very strong flavor, soak it for 30 minutes and discard the soaking water. Cook it in fresh water with seasonal land vegetables for about 45 minutes. For those unaccustomed to the taste, soak hijiki for 30 minutes and discard the water, then add fresh water and bring to boil for 1 minute, discard this water, add fresh water again, and then simmer for 45 minutes. To further enhance its taste, add sweet vegetables like onions, and season with wheat-free tamari. You can add apple juice toward the end of cooking, or use strong spices such as cayenne, chili powder, or curry, or seasonings like vinegar and garlic.

Agar-agar. *Use occasionally to make a kanten or aspic.* Agar-agar sea vegetable is a natural gelling agent that has a variety of culinary uses. It is available in flakes, bars, or powders for making jellies, aspics, or a kanten dessert. Add it to liquids like fruit juice or vegetable or bean broth, and simmer it until it dissolves. Then pour it into a desired mold, decorate with pieces of fruit if you wish, and let it set at room temperature for about one hour. You can create nice desserts in this way. See *Sweet Chocolaty Adzuki Bean Kanten* recipe in Step 9. For a strong bones soup, use one teaspoon of agar-agar to four cups of water.

Freshwater Algae. If you cannot eat sea vegetables, try freshwater blue-green algae like spirulina or chlorella powder as condiments or added to drinks to enhance the nutrient content of your meals. Algae contain the highest known levels of chlorophyll, which is vital for rapid assimilation of amino acids. Eating high-chlorophyll foods helps production of vitamin E in the body. These algae are known to assist peak performance of body, mind, and spirit and have found a place in detoxification or rejuvenation programs.[73] [74]

Recipes for Sea Vegetables from the Life-Giving Waters

Arame Sea Vegetable with Tempeh and Sauerkraut

4 servings

Arame is a nutrient-dense sea vegetable that is high in iron, calcium, zinc, and iodine and is also a rich source of lignans, which help fight cancer. The sweetness of arame combined with the heartiness of tempeh and the tang of sauerkraut gives this dish an interesting and pleasing texture and taste.

Ingredients:

½ cup arame sea vegetable
1 cup tempeh, cubed
2 tbsp. extra virgin olive oil or unrefined sesame oil
½ cup onion, sliced (optional)
1 cup sauerkraut, drained
Filtered or spring water to half cover dish
3 tbsp. tamari, or to taste
Garnish: scallions, finely sliced

Preparation:

1. Rinse, or soak the arame in cold water for 5 minutes, then drain and set aside.
2. Heat the oil in a frying pan and brown the tempeh cubes, tossing them around occasionally.
3. When tempeh is browned, add the onions, if using, and sauté them, adding a little water to prevent burning.
4. Add sauerkraut over tempeh and onions, and top it with the arame.
5. Half cover the dish with water and season with tamari. Bring to a quick boil, cover, lower the heat, and simmer for about 20 minutes.
6. Mix all, reseason if needed, and garnish with scallions. Serve with a grain and green leafy vegetable dish.

Variations:

- Omit sauerkraut and add a variety of seasonal vegetables like leeks, Chinese cabbage, carrots, or lotus root.
- Instead of tempeh, use tofu for another rich protein source.

Hijiki Sea Vegetable Delight with Corn and Broccoli

4 small side servings

Hijiki has one of the highest concentrations of calcium and iron of any food and is an excellent source of minerals and trace elements, as well as vitamins A, C, and B12. It has a strong flavor of the sea and a nutty aroma. Adding corn and broccoli makes a refreshing lighter salad.

Ingredients:

¼ cup hijiki sea vegetable
1 tbsp. unrefined light sesame oil
½ cup carrots or red onions, sliced
5 cloves garlic, minced (optional)
2 tbsp. tamari, or to taste
Filtered or spring water
1 cup yellow corn, fresh or frozen
1 cup broccoli florets
1 tbsp. lemon juice
Yellow or red pepper, cored and steamed (optional)
Garnish: scallions or parsley, finely chopped

Preparation:

1. Rinse and soak the hijiki in cold water for 20 minutes (it will double in size).
2. Drain, cut into smaller pieces, and set aside.
3. Heat a stainless steel skillet; add oil, sauté onions or carrots and garlic (if using) for 1 minute.
4. Add hijiki and 1 tbsp. of tamari and briefly sauté.
5. Add water to half cover the dish. Bring to a quick boil, then lower heat and cover.
6. Simmer between 30 and 45 minutes. Toward the end, add the corn and broccoli, reseason with the rest of the tamari, drizzle lemon juice over the dish, and mix.
7. Optionally, serve in a steamed pepper for color, and garnish with fresh scallions or parsley.
8. Use long grain rice and a bean and a vegetable dish to complement the meal.

Variations:

• Instead of hijiki, use arame sea vegetable.
• Occasionally serve hijiki combined with root vegetables like lotus root, fried tofu, or tempeh, to make a strong cold weather dish.
• Season with your favorite herbs and spices, or add sweet rice miso for a lighter dish.
• Hijiki can be cooked longer, 1¼ to 1½ hours total cooking time, and it becomes sweeter.

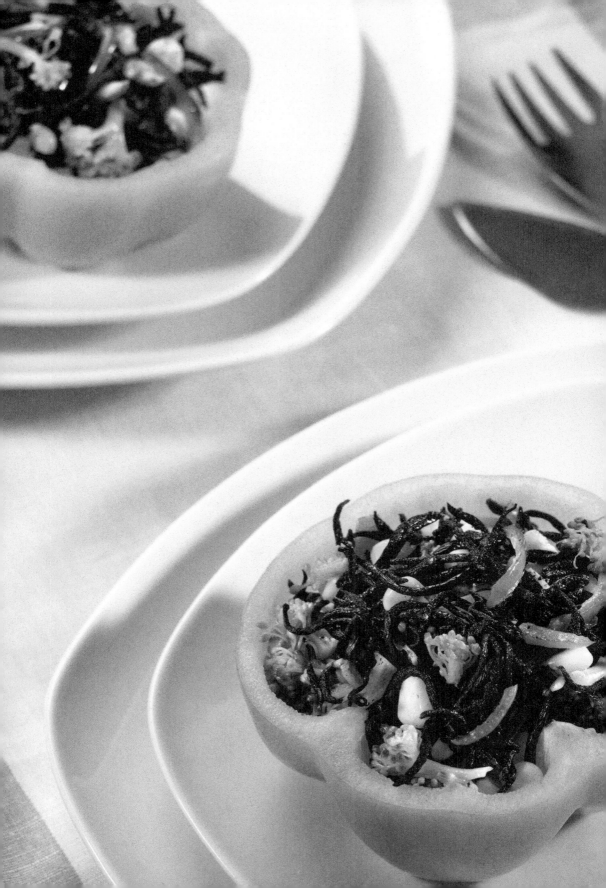

Fresh Wakame Sea Vegetable Salad with Kale

3 side servings

Wakame contains cleansing and fat-eliminating nutrients. It is low in saturated fat and very low in cholesterol, and contains many vitamins, minerals and other health-supportive nutrients. Wakame is very high in sodium, so always soak (or rinse) before using and discard the soaking water.

Ingredients:
2 cups kale
1/3 cup wakame sea vegetable strands
1–2 scallions or parsley, finely sliced
Seasoning:
1 tbsp. tamari, or to taste
2 tbsp. umeboshi vinegar, or to taste
Drizzles of roasted sesame oil, or to taste
Toasted brown sesame seeds

Preparation:
1. Wash kale and remove the spine, then mince very finely.
2. Soak wakame strands in water for 5 minutes. Drain.
3. Remove inner harder vein (set aside for other dishes), and slice the strands.
4. Combine greens and wakame with scallions in a large bowl.
5. Add seasonings and mix. You can press the salad or just let sit for half an hour before serving.
6. Serve as a side dish with grain, bean, and vegetable dishes.

Variations:
•   Use instant wakame flakes, these have the harder vein already removed.
•   Use cucumber instead of kale.
•   Instead of umeboshi vinegar, use lemon juice to taste.

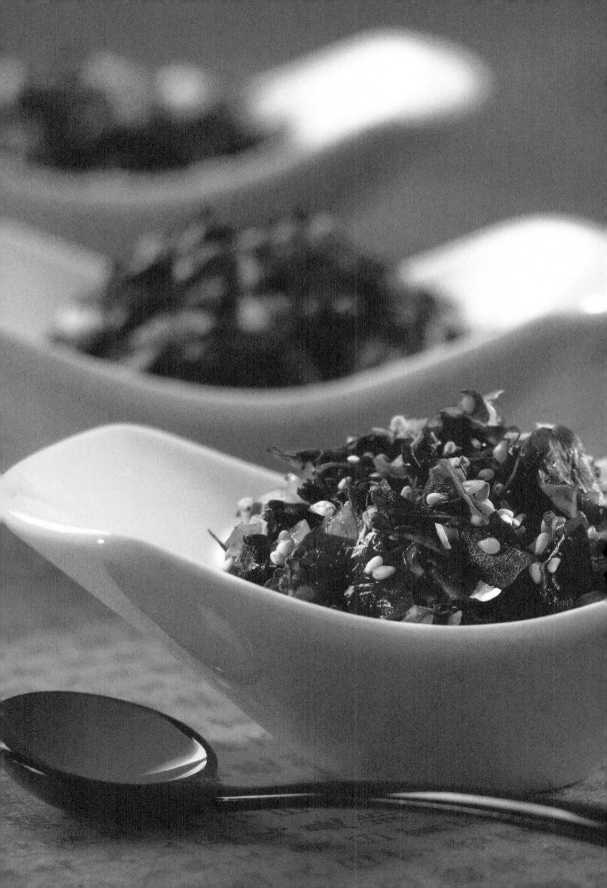

Sea Vegetable Roll with Tofu And Carrots

4 servings

All sea vegetables are traditionally valued for their natural mineral content and ability to enrich and cleanse the blood. Adding tofu and carrots to a quick-cooking sea vegetable like arame makes a well-rounded dish that is a welcome addition to your menu.

Ingredients:

¼ cup arame sea vegetable
1 tbsp. unrefined sesame oil
1 cup onions, sliced (optional)
1 cup carrot, matchsticks
1 cup tofu, cubed
Filtered or spring water
2 tbsp. tamari, or to taste
2 tsp. umeboshi vinegar
Few drops lemon juice, or to taste; 1 sheet nori
Garnish inside the rolls: parsley or ingredients of your choice
Dip: tamari, water, and wasabi (Japanese horseradish), to taste

Preparation:

1. Rinse and soak the arame in cold water for 5 minutes and drain.
2. Brush skillet with small amount of sesame oil. Add the onions, if using, and carrots and sauté for 2 minutes.
3. Layer the tofu, followed by the arame, on top of the vegetables.
4. Add water to cover up to the level of the arame.
5. Add about 1 tbsp. tamari and 1 tsp. umeboshi vinegar, bring to a boil, cover, and simmer on medium low for about 15 minutes. Add water if necessary.
6. Season with rest of the tamari and umeboshi vinegar to taste, and simmer until all the remaining liquid is gone.
7. Add a few drops of lemon juice. (At this point you also have a dish that can be served as is.)
8. To make the roll, squeeze out and drain any remaining liquids from the cooked arame.
9. On a bamboo sushi mat (or use a cutting board and roll by hand), place one sheet of toasted nori.
10. Place the drained arame ½ inch thick on the nori, leaving 1 inch on the top and bottom.
11. Spread parsley or garnishes of your choice evenly in a line in the middle of the arame.
12. Start lifting the sushi mat, (or use your hands) and press and tuck the arame into the nori.
13. Roll the dish into a cylinder, press and tuck arame into the nori as you lift.
14. At the end, wet the edges of the nori with a bit of water and press together so it sticks.
15. Cut the roll into even pieces. Arrange them on a serving platter, and serve with a dip.

Variations:

• Use other vegetable like leeks, Chinese (Napa) cabbage, or lotus root.

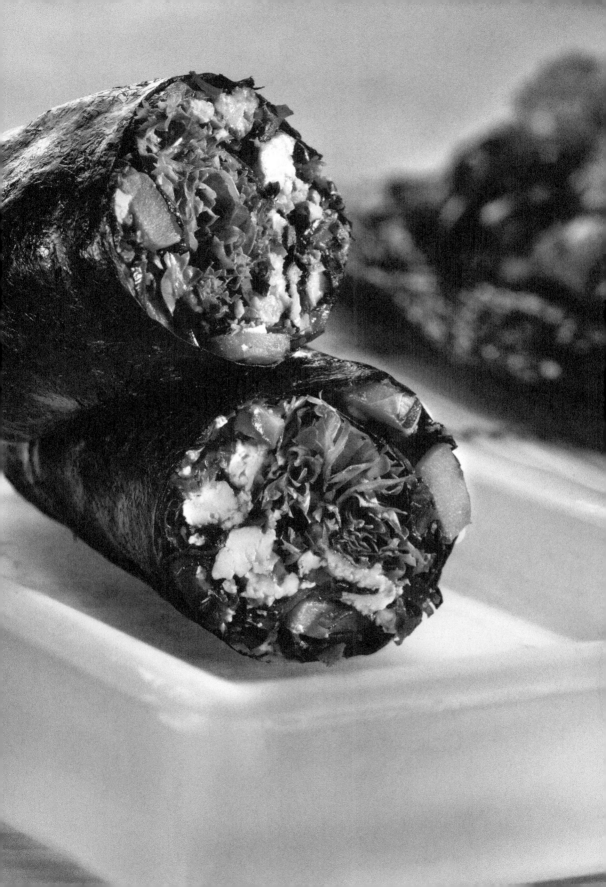

Cauliflower and Sea Vegetables Curry

4 servings

This dish adds Indian spices to European land vegetables and Oriental sea vegetables. It is a fun way to combine many nutrients from different cultures and a welcome variation when eating sea vegetables. This is the perfect dish to enjoy during hot weather.

Ingredients:

1 tbsp. coconut oil
½ cup onions, minced (optional)
Pinch sea salt
1 cup arame sea vegetable
2+ cups cauliflower, cut into florets
1 cup green peas
1 can light coconut milk
2 tsp. curry powder, or to taste
2 tsp. tamari, or to taste
≈ 1 tsp. balsamic vinegar
Garnish: cilantro sprigs

Preparation:

1. Rinse arame and soak in cold water 5–10 minutes. Drain and set aside.
2. Heat oil in a deep frying pan and sauté onions till translucent. Add sea salt and stir.
3. Add arame, cauliflower, and peas.
4. Add coconut milk, saving some to use at the end of cooking.
5. Mix in curry, tamari, and vinegar and stir.
6. Bring to a quick boil, cover, lower the heat, and simmer for 15 minutes, or till cauliflower is soft.
7. Reseason if needed, and add the saved coconut milk to freshen the taste.
8. Serve over long grain basmati or short grain brown rice, garnished with cilantro.

Variations:

- Use half water-half coconut milk for a lighter taste.
- Omit coconut milk and use only water, or other varieties of non-dairy milk.
- Add diced sweet potato to the vegetable mix.
- Use chickpeas for added protein and taste.

Breakfast or any time dishes

Nori –Toasted or Raw

Eating sea vegetables for breakfast is easier then you think. Eat half or an entire sheet of nori for breakfast. Just nibbling on a toasted or raw sheet of nori is all you need to start the day right with minerals and vitamins. For already-toasted nori, get the sushi variety.

Soft Nori Condiment

Adding a nori condiment as a salty topping on your morning grain porridge is another great way to include sea vegetables for breakfast. Use this condiment for any other meal as a flavor and nutrient boost.

Ingredients:
4 nori sheets
¼ cup filtered or spring water
Tamari, to taste

Preparation:
1. Shred several sheets of raw or toasted nori into small pieces and place in a pan.
2. Gently add water to half cover the nori and bring to a quick boil, then simmer and stir gently until all the pieces are dissolved.
3. Add tamari to taste. Serve as a condiment with a grain or noodle dish.
4. Store in the refrigerator for about 5 days.

Variations:
• Add other seasonings towards the end like mirin, minced scallions, ginger juice, or finely grated garlic for a change in taste.

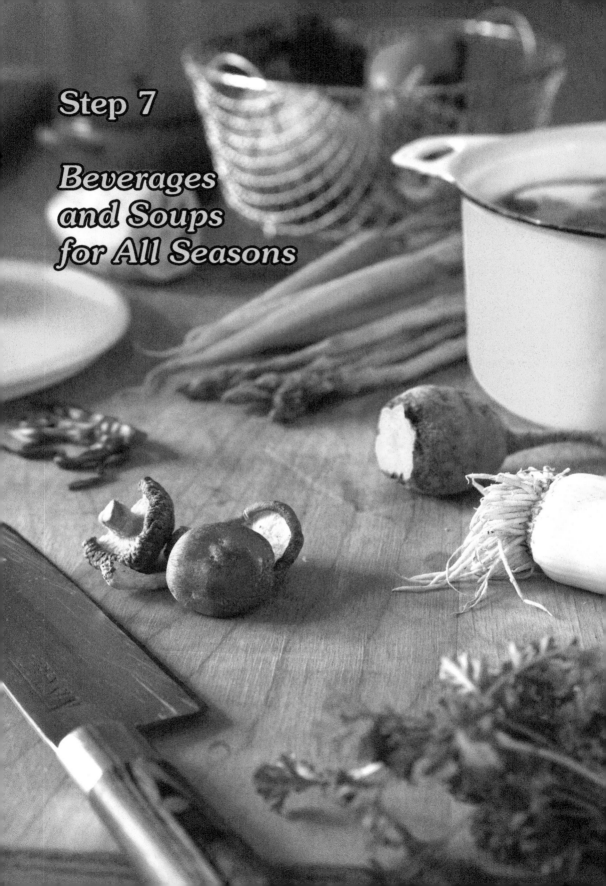

Step 7

Beverages
and Soups
for All Seasons

You have many beverages or soups to choose from, and all these liquid forms of nourishment have one thing in common—they all contain water. Water is the basis of all life, and that includes your body. At birth, a baby's body is about 90% water. An adult body contains about 70% water. Our body's water content can drop as much as 50% with age. The muscles that move your body are 75% water; your blood that transports nutrients is 82% water; your lungs that provide your oxygen are 90% water; your brain that is the control center of your body is 76% water; and even your bones are 25% water. Our health is truly dependent on the quality and quantity of the water we drink.[75]

Liquids: How Much We Need to Rehydrate and Cleanse

How do you start your day? Is a cup of coffee or tea your favorite beverage to break your fast? Rehydrating in the morning with a cup of water before drinking anything else or eating breakfast is one of the best ways to start your day. Drink it hot or at room temperature, and if you like the taste, add a twist of lemon. Water will replenish the liquid you used during the night and will flush out toxins in your body.

During the day, between meals, use it as replacement for other beverages, especially sodas or soft drinks. All sodas have tremendous amounts of sugar, and drinking these regularly can add to the risk of diabetes and weight gain. Diet sodas have artificial sweeteners that are best avoided. Avoid or limit using ice water, water with ice cubes, or any ice-cold beverages or soups, as the ice will temporarily freeze, or slow down, your digestive system and hinder the absorption of your food. Some say that is a great way to lose weight, yet it's a very unhealthy one, as you don't absorb any nutrients at all. Of course, sometimes a refreshing cold drink is just what you need to relax on a hot summer day.

Your water intake can vary depending on the season and climate zone you live in, and your age, activity level, goals in life, and gender. Your daily hydration need increases when you spend time in air-conditioned rooms, exercise, take part in sports, do heavy work, undergo medical treatment, take vitamins, have increased sun exposure, or sweat. Consider also increasing your skin care with organic and vegan moisturizing creams.

Some say that when you are feeling thirsty, your body is already lacking liquid. Watch your salt intake, as too much salt can make you thirstier. Having too many liquids in relation to your solid food intake can also bring you out of balance. Some even say that drinking too much liquid can actually kill you. Where do you draw the line, and what kind of beverage is the right one for you? Scientists are still arguing about how much water an adult person should drink. The numbers range from 1.5 to 2 liters (4 to 8 eight-ounce cups) of liquid as a recommended daily amount. Do your own research and talk to your physician to make sure you drink the right amount of liquid for your needs, especially if you are doing out-of-the-ordinary activities, as either excessive or not enough liquid can weaken your system.

Many people do not have access to clean drinking water, and many others are unhappy about the taste and smell of their tap water. If you use tap water for drinking and cooking, you might want to purify or filter it, starting with a good carbon water filter, or get your water containers filled from local certified clean spring or well water sources. For further health benefits, consider alkaline electron-rich water or ionized water.[76]

Avoid plastic water bottles, as these may pose health risks from chemicals in the plastics; they also definitely pollute the landscape. Use your own sustainable containers, such as glass or stainless steel bottles. Buy environmentally friendly products, and avoid discarding hazardous household products or medications down the sink or toilet, as this contaminates the water supply.[77] You might also consider supporting clean water sourcing for the Third World. These are easy steps toward a sustainable lifestyle.

Since you cook with water, drink soups and other beverages, and eat stews, dressings, and sauces, you obtain some of your daily hydration from these sources. Before your meals, have a small bowl of soup that is lightly seasoned with fermented miso paste, with its beneficial enzymes. This can help you to digest your food and provides you with liquid. See Step 5 for further information on miso.

Drinking a glass of water with your meals can dilute your digestive enzymes. Instead, drink water between your meals for better digestion and to detoxify. Water consumed between meals will very quickly pass through the stomach and the GI tract.

Beverage Considerations: History and Health Factors

People have been brewing leaves, sticks, fruits, flowers, roots, bark, and berries for centuries. Gather your own materials and brew these caffeine-free teas according to your needs, or look for them in your stores. Note that yerba mate, kola nut, and guarana contain caffeine.

Everyday Teas

Try *kukicha* twig tea or *bancha*, the roasted stems or leaves of the mature green tea plant. Kukicha and bancha ("kuki" means twig and "cha" means tea in Japanese) have digestion-calming and alkaline properties. Kukicha and bancha can be used daily. Drink them hot, cold, plain, or mixed with apple juice in the summer. The leaves and stems can be purchased loose and brewed for the desired strength and can often be used at least twice. A darker golden color indicates a stronger, more yang energy, and is good to use in the cold season or when feeling weak. A light golden brew might be preferred in hot weather. Kukicha has a small amount of caffeine, similar to decaffeinated teas, and some say it also has a better taste. Decaffeinated teas often have a chemical residue from the decaffeinating process. One study showed that residues of a known carcinogen, methylene chloride, were 400 percent higher in decaffeinated tea than even in decaffeinated coffee. Use kukicha tea instead of decaffeinated coffee or tea when you wish to regulate your caffeine intake. For home remedies and tonics with kukicha, see Step 10. You can also take kukicha teabags with you on the road, and use them in restaurants, at work, or when you travel.

Kukicha Preparation: Place 1½ to 2 tablespoons of roasted twigs in 1½ quarts of water and bring to a boil. For a darker tea, simmer 5–10 minutes. For a lighter tea, simmer 2–3 minutes. Strain and reuse the twigs.

Green Teas

Green teas have important antioxidants and compounds that are known for their health benefits. In the East, where green tea is a dietary mainstay, large-scale human studies have found that green tea has shown a promising impact on heart disease and cancer, although other Eastern lifestyle factors might also have had a strong effect on the outcome of the studies.[78] Green tea has caffeine and is more yin than the roasted kukicha or bancha. Green tea with roasted brown rice, available in tea bags and loose, is also a good choice as a beverage. Adding a twist of lemon juice to your green tea can maximize the antioxidant power in your cup.[79]

Grain Teas

Roasted grains like rice brewed with an ample amount of water also provide a tasty drink for adults and children alike.

Digestive, Immune-Enhancing, Relaxing and Stimulating Herbal Teas

To make a digestive tea, add grated ginger juice and mint to water and boil, or use kombucha, a fermented tea. To stimulate your immune response, include ginseng, peppermint, and echinacea.

Relaxing teas and herbal bedtime blends can contain chamomile, hops, linden flowers, lavender, passionflower, skullcap, valerian, tilia buds, or white zapote. *Kava kava*, a South Pacific tea, also relaxes tense muscles. Teas made with stimulating spices such as cardamom, cinnamon, vanilla, and ginger root will warm you internally and fuel your digestion and elimination. These herbs or spices need to brew for about ten minutes to bring out their distinct flavor. For specific macrobiotic tea home remedies, see Step 10.

Alcoholic Beverages

It goes without saying that alcoholic beverages should be drunk responsibly and age-appropriately. Since drinking any kind of alcoholic beverage dehydrates your system, drink a glass of water with it. Use alcohol on social occasions only, and when your health permits. Digestion-stimulating spices like cardamom, cinnamon, and ginger, and also berries, can be added to some alcoholic beverages as one-week infusions. Before serving, mix these infusions with kombucha tea or rejuvelac, both fermented liquids, and water, plus optional ice if needed. Serve these alcohol-reduced options as cleansing beverages on social occasions, if health permits.

Beer, in Teutonic and other northern European traditions, was a daily lactic acid-containing fermented drink with very little alcohol in it. It served as a kind of "miso soup," a digestive helper (more yin, however, than actual miso soup.) Various folk groups in northern Europe at one time all had their special roots and herbs for prolonging the life of beer, which also gave a very typical taste for each one. Experiment with mixing beer, preferably organic, unfiltered, and naturally brewed, with freshly pressed juices, unsweetened, unfiltered, and not from concentrate. In this way you can reduce the alcohol percentage. Here are some interesting possibilities.

1. To ¼–½ glass of pure unfiltered apple juice, add ½–¾ glass of organic beer (unfiltered, if possible). This is a very refreshing drink on hot summer evenings. Light beer works the best here.
2. To ¼–½ glass of pure unsweetened red fruit juice (mixed fruits like red grapes, sweet red cherries, red currants, raspberries, or other northern red fruits), add ½–¾ glass of beer. This is refreshing in the cooler season and carries lots of antioxidants. Works with both light and dark beer.

3. Add ¼–½ glass of blackberry, blueberry, morello cherry, or other blue or black fruit juice to ½–¾ glass of beer. A refreshing warm-season drink with light beer, and cold-season drink with dark beer.

Variations:

*   Instead of fruit juice, add a small amount of rejuvelac (less than 1/8 glass, as it has a strongly sour taste). Healthy lactic acid is normally found in naturally brewed beer, but rejuvelac allows you to increase the lactic acid content. Experiment with various mixtures according to your personal needs and preferred tastes, and health permitting.

Gluten Advice: most beers and alcoholic beverages contain gluten.

What Kind of Beverages to Drink and When

Daily Use
*   Filtered, purified, or spring water
*   Kukicha twig tea, loose or in tea bags
*   Bancha leaf tea, loose or in tea bags
*   Roasted rice tea: roast grain in pan; boil with water to desired strength.
*   Roasted brown rice with green tea, loose or in tea bags

Occasional Use
*   Grain coffee (100% grain, may contain gluten)
*   Dandelion tea
*   Kombu tea: boil kombu in water for 10 minutes
*   Umeboshi tea: boil water and umeboshi plum for 10 minutes
*   Mu tea
*   Carrot juice, celery juice, vegetable juice blend, green drink
*   Sweet vegetable drink (recipe in Step 10)
*   Stimulant herb teas
*   Kombucha tea (fermented drink)
*   Green tea
*   Fruit juice, homemade or purchased
*   Soymilk (with kombu), rice milk, almond milk, or other nut milk
*   Barley sprouts powder (contains gluten), spirulina, and chlorella

Infrequent Use or Social Occasions
*   Mineralized water
*   Carbonated sparkling water
*   Coffee
*   Most black teas
*   Sake (hot or cold)
*   Wine

- Beer
- Whiskey (on rare occasions, health permitting)
- Herb-infused alcoholic beverages
- Iced drinks (with ice cubes)

Avoid
- Hard liquors
- Sugared and soft drinks
- Commercial teas (with caffeine, decaffeinated, or chemically colored)
- Sodas or other stimulant aromatic sugar beverages
- Distilled water

Water—And Your Way of Life

One of the central macrobiotic lifestyle concepts is that our daily meals should mirror our evolutionary development. At mealtime, start with a soup that contains a small amount of sea vegetables, sea salt, or fermented foods like miso and tamari. A soup prepared in this way represents the conditions of life's early development on earth and brings us in contact with our evolution.

A natural way of living is drinking when you are thirsty, eating when you are hungry, and sleeping when you are tired. Get in the habit of drinking your water and other beverages slowly, and pause for several seconds before swallowing. Don't allow large swallows. Drink your beverages hot or at room temperature. Avoid drinks right out of the refrigerator. Take them out and let them sit awhile. Don't use ice-cold drinks.

Sip your beverages and soups and mix them with saliva in order to digest them properly. Solid foods should be chewed at least 30–40 times per mouthful to liquefy them—or even longer, up to one hundred times, especially when attempting to heal your body. When you chew your food, the enzyme amylase is activated in your mouth, which helps break down your food and aids absorption.

More chewing might also be a good way to eat less food, as researchers suspect that the mere act of chewing switches on your brain's satiety center. In one study, forty chews of the same amount of nuts helped curb hunger better than ten or twenty chews, and the feeling of fullness lasted longer.[80] Try this for yourself, as this practice may work with other foods too.

Beverage sizes have grown, and the amount we eat has also increased, so we tend to overeat. Counteract the bigger-is-better motto. Ask in restaurants for smaller servings, use smaller cups and glasses for your drinks, and serve soups in small cups or small bowls.

Dr. Masaru Emoto, author of The Miracle of Water and many other books, says that water has healing powers on its own.[81] His studies further show that water crystals are influenced by energy. Placing your hands over your food and giving thanks for the food and water you use daily could have an influence on the energetics of your meals.

History of Soups

Combining nutritious grains, beans, and vegetables and cooking them in a pot of water is one of the easiest ways to provide a quick meal. Soups are one of the first foods that people made when they discovered cooking. Locally available foods and tastes have dictated the ingredients of all the popular soups and stews. Russian borscht, Italian minestrone, Spanish gazpacho, French onion soup and bouillon, Chinese wonton soup, Japanese miso soups, and German vegetable, legume, sausage, and potato stews—all have found recognition in the culinary world.

Soups with herbs and vegetables also have been greatly valued since ancient times as healing agents. Chicken noodle soup still holds first place in many cultures as a curative concoction, and friends often advise it when cold season is upon us. For a warm, comforting vegan hot beverage, try a Japanese dashi made with kombu, shiitake, and miso. Drinking a cup of miso soup a day may keep the doctor away.

The word *soup* is derived from "sop" or "sup," which refers to a slice of bread on which the broth was poured. Before bread, people used gruel grains to make thick stews. Soups were the first food served in public restaurants in Paris in the eighteenth century. Clear soups like broth, bouillon, and consommé are important in classic French cuisine. The word *restaurant* comes from an Old French variant of "restorative," which is associated with a medicine or drink that restores health.

Scientific advancements have brought us many forms of portable soups, from canned and dehydrated to microwave-ready, for specific dietary needs ranging from low salt to high fiber to gluten-free. You might have some of your own favorite soups in one of these forms. Hopefully this Step will provide you with ideas that allow you to easily make your own soups that are more nutritious then any of these. When you travel, however, some form of portable soup might be helpful in staying with your goals.

Seasonal Reflections on Soups and Healthy Considerations

The nutrient content of your soups, dressings, and sauces depends on the soup stock and the herbs, spices, seasonings, and other ingredients you add to it. Soups, sauces, and dressings can be eaten in all seasons, and the ingredients should reflect the season. Choose ingredients for your soups and stews from the seasonal charts of the previous Steps. Keep it simple! Use what you have at hand.

In warmer months, seasonings, dressings, and sauces can be very light. Green vegetable soups are delicious fare for the spring season. A clear broth, French onion soup, or yellow lentil soup are energizing in late summer. Some of your favorite soups that taste great hot can also make an interesting room temperature or cold soup during hotter weather.[82] Experiment with a cold fruit soup or a cold miso soup for a refreshing treat.

During fall and winter, try preparations according to your needs with more or less liquid, salt, oil, and miso. Eat hot soups made with root and round vegetables such as squash. Whole grain and bean stews provide great energy in colder weather.

Remember that in any season, drinking too much liquid or eating too many soups in relation to your other food intake and activities can bring you out of balance—you might deplete the energy of the kidney and bladder.

Making Dashi, Broth, and Stocks for Soups, Dressings, and Sauces

Start by making flavorful vegetable stocks or a kombu-shiitake mushroom dashi, and have them on hand. Most soup and stew recipes call for beef, chicken, or fish stock. Therefore having a variety of delicious-tasting land vegetable, sea vegetable, or mushroom stocks on hand gives you greater flexibility in your plant-centered kitchen.

You do not need to start with whole vegetables—you can use organic vegetable scraps and peelings. Instead of tossing or composting the cores of cauliflower or cabbage, parsley stems, organic squash or carrot skins, or other vegetable and mushroom ends, dedicate one container in your kitchen for saving them for making vegetable stock. You can freeze leftover stock in ice cube trays. Store the cubes in a dated glass container to defrost and use as needed. If you choose to make an animal stock, we recommend the use of bones and heads of land or water animals instead of the flesh.

Recipes for Beverages and Soups
for All Seasons

Miso Soups for All Seasons and Reasons
4 servings

A well-prepared miso soup enriches intestinal flora and supports immunity, and thus is good in all seasons. Miso has a nutritious balance of carbohydrates, essential oils (no cholesterol), vitamins, minerals like calcium, and protein. Use long time fermented brown (red) rice miso, soybean miso, or barley miso (contains gluten) year round, but especially during colder weather or in a healing soup. Enjoy short time fermented mellow rice or chickpea miso that are less salty more often during the warmer seasons. Mixing the different flavors of miso can have interesting results.

Ingredients:
2–3 dried shiitake mushrooms
6-inch piece kombu sea vegetable
4 cups filtered or spring water
½ cup onions, diced
2 cups daikon radish, diced
½ cake tofu, small cubes
2 tsp. instant wakame flakes, quickly rinsed
4 tsp. brown rice miso, diluted in warm broth
Garnish: sliced scallions

Preparation:
1. Soak shiitake mushroom and kombu for 10 minutes in 4 cups of water.
2. Bring all to a quick boil and simmer for 10 minutes.
3. Remove kombu and save for another dish.
4. Slice shiitake mushroom, discard stems, and put the slices back into the water.
5. Add onions, daikon, and tofu to the broth. Bring to a boil and simmer until all is soft.
6. Add instant wakame flakes and diluted miso.
7. Stir and gently low simmer for 3 to 5 minutes, being careful not to boil the soup.
8. Serve hot and garnish with scallions.

Variations:
• Instead of instant wakame flakes, use whole wakame strands, soaked 5 minutes and sliced.
• Use any combination of seasonal vegetables.
• Add cooked grains like millet or beans like lentils.
• Choose different miso flavors, or mix and match them.
• Add umeboshi paste for added flavor.
• Use sweet rice mirin for a sweet-flavored miso soup.

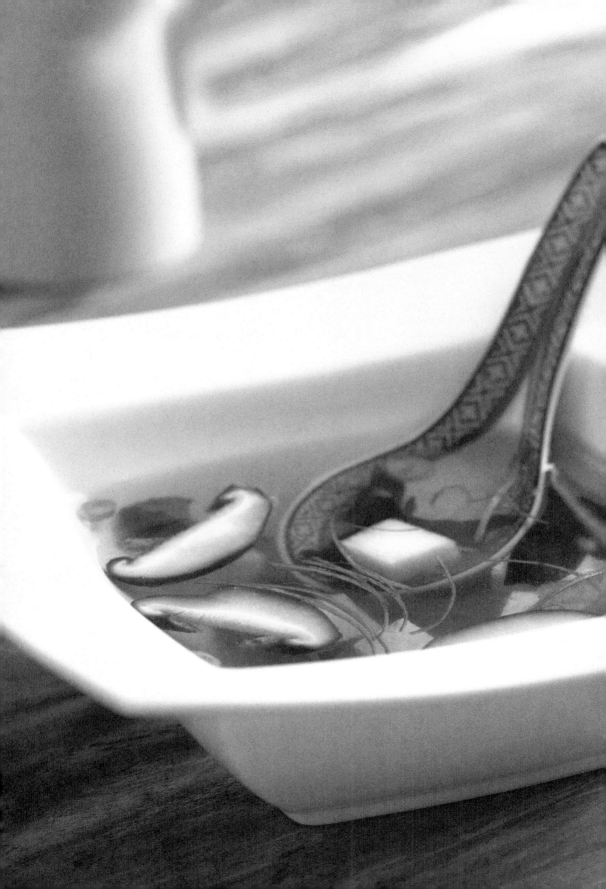

Gluten-Conscious Noodle Soup

4 servings

This wonderful soup is a great substitute for wheat noodle soups. Try quinoa, corn, brown rice, buckwheat, or rice noodles, or mung bean vermicelli. Choose between different shapes of noodles like spirals, ribbons, or strands. All work well.

Ingredients:

1-inch strip kombu
2 dried shiitake mushrooms
4 cups filtered or spring water
½ cup onions, sliced thin (optional)
1 cup carrots, cut julienne style
1 cup gluten-free noodles
4 tsp. miso of your choice, diluted in warm water
1 cup snow peas, cut into strips (leave some for garnish)
Fresh grated ginger or its juice, to taste
Garnish: sliced scallions and snow peas

Preparation:

1. Prepare soup stock with kombu and shiitake by first soaking for 10 minutes in water and then boiling 10 minutes.
2. Remove kombu. Discard stems of mushrooms, slice the caps, and add back to the pot.
3. Add onions, if using, and carrots. Bring to a boil and simmer until the vegetables are nearly done, yet still crunchy.
4. Meanwhile, cook noodles in a separate pot of water until still hard in the center.
5. Drain noodles and rinse with cold water.
6. Add the noodles and snow peas to the pot of vegetables and broth.
7. Add diluted miso and simmer on low flame for 3-5 minutes; don't boil.
8. Add fresh ginger to taste, stir, garnish, and serve in individual bowls.

Variations:

- Use a different soup stock, or other seasonal vegetables.
- Omit miso; use tamari, or season with sea salt, black pepper, and herbs of your choice.
- Add greens like chopped watercress at the end of cooking. Add beans or tofu.

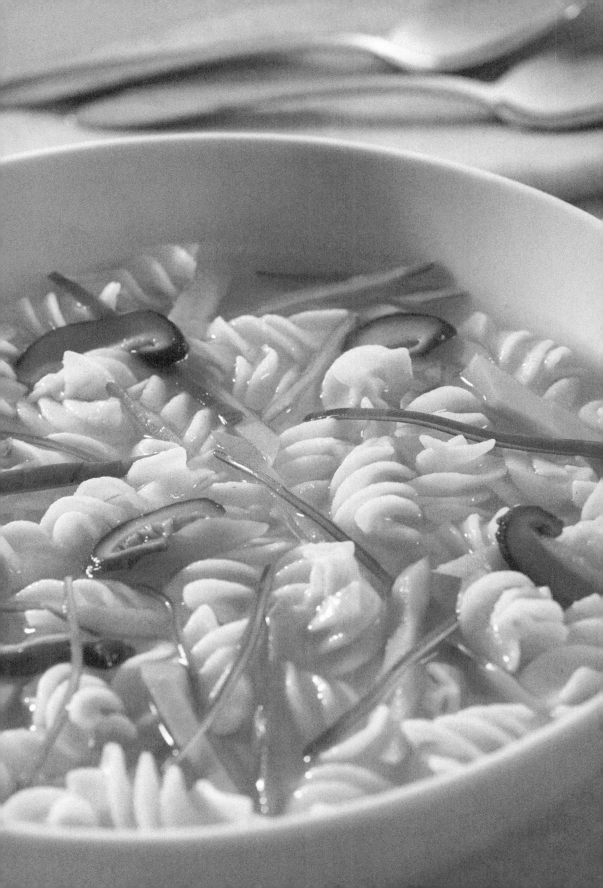

Summer's Sweetest Native Traditions

4 servings

Several Native American tribes traditionally grew sweet corn, and the Iroquois gave the first recorded sweet corn to European settlers in the year 1779.[83] Nowadays corn is very popular and eaten around the world. Cooking sweet corn activates its antioxidants, which are known to reduce the chance of heart disease and cancer. Choose organic, non-GMO corn.

Ingredients:

1 large white onion, minced
1 tsp. high-oleic safflower oil
Kernels sliced from 4 cobs of corn
4–6 cups filtered or spring water
4–6 tsp. sweet rice miso, diluted with warm broth
Dash of umeboshi vinegar
Garnish: sliced scallions or parsley, nori strips, or finely sliced kale

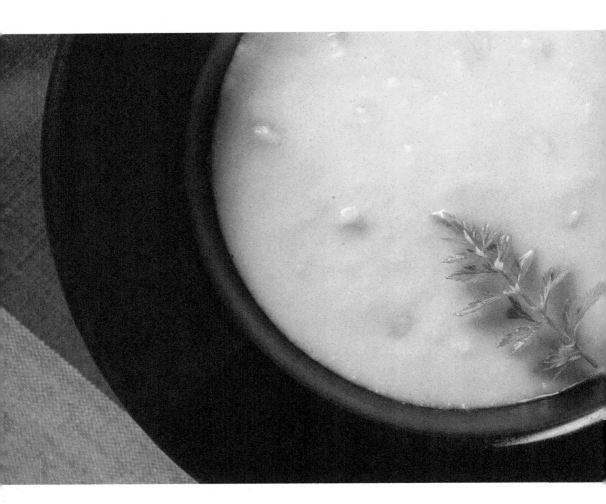

Preparation:
1. Heat oil on medium high in a large pot and sauté onions until translucent.
2. Add corn and water and bring to a boil, then simmer for 20 minutes.
3. Optional: puree half the corn with a handheld blender.
4. Add diluted miso and a dash of vinegar, and simmer for 5 minutes.
5. Serve hot and garnish. Bring umeboshi vinegar to the table to add more if desired.

Variations:
- Add carrots, celery, and other summer vegetables.
- Use frozen or canned corn (unsweetened).
- Use half water/half non-dairy milk.
- Use red wine vinegar instead of umeboshi vinegar.
- If the stew is too soupy, thicken with a kuzu/cold water mix in the proportion 1 tsp. kuzu per 1 cup of liquid.

Vegetable Stock with Herbs

5 servings

Making your own stock is easy. Using your favorite land or water vegetables and herbs to bring out the flavors you like best is definitely worth the small effort. This stock is an excellent base for creating tasty sauces, risotto, soups, stews, or any savory plant-based dish that calls for liquid.

Vegetable ingredients:
2 leeks, white and green part, sliced
4 medium onions, big chunks with skin (optional)
6 large carrots, big chunks
1 large celery root, diced
3 celery stalks, including the heart and the leaves, sliced
6 cups cold filtered or spring water
1 bunch parsley, with stems
½ tsp. sea salt

Herbal mix:
1 tsp. dried marjoram
½ tsp. dried thyme
3 small bay leaves
12 peppercorns, or to taste
3 large garlic cloves, or to taste

Preparation:
1. Place washed and chopped leeks, onions, carrots, celery root, celery stalks, and parsley in a large pot and cover with water, about 6 cups.
2. Stir in herbal mix and salt. Bring to a boil, reduce heat, cover, and simmer for at least one hour.

3. Strain the stock through a fine strainer, and press the vegetables to extract all liquid.
4. Compost the leftover vegetables. Broth keeps in the fridge for about three days.
5. Freeze leftover stock in ice cube trays, then store in a freezer container and date. Add to stews, soups, sauces, and dips as needed.

Variations:

*   Roast vegetables in a 350° F oven for 30 minutes or stir-fry before placing in the pot.
*   Caramelize the onions by sautéing them in olive oil before adding them to the broth.
*   Add kombu, mushrooms, ginger, or your favorite vegetables.
*   Add leftover vegetable peels.

Pressure-Cooked Kidney Bean Stew with Squash and Carrots

4 servings

Few things are more inviting to come home to on a freezing winter day than a steaming pot of beans, fragrant with seasonings and hearty vegetables. One-dish meals like this are perfect for cold-season or anytime lunches, perhaps with a slice of sourdough whole grain bread and some pickles on the side.

Ingredients:

1 cup kidney beans
3–5 cups filtered or spring water
1-inch piece kombu sea vegetable
¼ tsp. sea salt
1/3 cup onions, diced (optional)
1/3 cup carrots, diced
1/3 cup squash, diced
2–4 tsp. dark rice miso, diluted in warm water
1 tbsp. tahini
1 clove garlic, pressed (optional)
1 tsp. arrowroot or kuzu, diluted in cold water (optional)
Garnish: scallions or parsley, sliced

Preparation:

1. Soak beans to cover in 3–5 cups water for eight hours or overnight. Rinse kombu.
2. Discard bean-soaking water and replace with about 3 cups of fresh water.
3. Place kombu, beans, and water in the pressure cooker and bring to a boil. Remove any foam that may rise to the surface and replace the water you scooped out.
4. Close the lid and pressure cook 45 minutes or according to your pressure cooker timetable. (If boiling in a regular pot, it takes about 2 hours.)

5. Allow the pressure to come completely down. Open the pot and optional remove kombu.
6. Season with sea salt, stir, and layer the onions (if using), carrots, and squash on top of the beans.
7. Bring to a quick boil, and then simmer until vegetables are soft. Don't pressure-cook at this point.
8. If too soupy, thicken with arrowroot or kuzu /cold water mix, in the proportion 1 tsp. of arrowroot or kuzu per 1 cup of soup liquid.
9. Add miso, tahini, and, if using, garlic, and simmer on low for about 5 minutes.
10. Serve in individual bowls and garnish with finely sliced scallions or parsley.

Variations:

- Use black turtle beans, split peas, or adzuki.
- Cook extra beans and set some aside for other dishes.

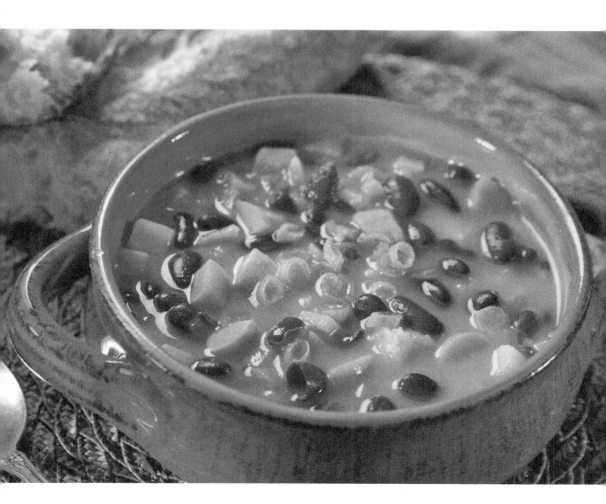

Strengthening Kimpira Root Vegetable Soup

4 servings

Burdock and carrots are the main ingredients in the vegetable side dish kimpira. In this strengthening soup, we add a variety of other root and round vegetables. Depending on the season and your needs, add dandelion or omit another root.

Ingredients:

1 tsp. light unrefined sesame oil
½ cup onions, chopped (optional)
¾ cup burdock, julienne style
¾ cup carrots, julienne style
½ cup lotus root, julienne style
½ cup winter squash, finely cubed
Pinch sea salt
5 cups filtered or spring water, or soup stock
½ cup green leafy vegetables, finely sliced
1 tbsp. dark rice miso, diluted with warm water
1 tbsp. sweet miso, diluted with warm water
Garnish: finely sliced scallions

Preparation:

1. Lightly brush skillet with sesame oil and heat. First sauté the onions, if using, until light brown, then add the root vegetables and sauté for 2– 3 minutes, and finally the squash.
2. Add sea salt and cover vegetables with water or soup stock and simmer for about 20 minutes.
3. When all vegetables are soft, add the rest of the water, if wanted.
4. Add any finely sliced green leafy vegetable you have on hand.
5. Add the miso to the soup. Simmer for 5 minutes on low heat.
6. Garnish individual bowls of soup with finely sliced scallions.

Variations:

- Use a teaspoon or so of dark sesame oil toward the end of cooking to give a strong taste.
- Omit miso and season with your favorite spices or herbs.
- If fresh lotus root is not available, use the dried root and soak before adding to the soup.
- Add diced green cabbage to the mix.

Mediterranean Garbanzo Soup

4 servings

This hearty soup is a welcome late summer and autumn delight. Garbanzo beans (chickpeas) are delicious legumes that provide great protein, and their high amounts of insoluble fiber and antioxidants help to regulate cholesterol and lower the risk of colon cancer. Cook extra chickpeas and make hummus by mashing chickpeas, garlic, tahini, lemon and olive oil until smooth.

Ingredients:

2 cups dried garbanzos
5 cups filtered or spring water or Herbal Vegetable Stock (see above)
1-2 bay leaves
¼ tsp. sea salt
1 tbsp. extra virgin olive oil
1 cup onions, diced (optional)
1 tbsp. garlic, crushed (optional)
1 cup carrots, diced
1-2 stalks celery, diced
½-1 cup celery root, diced
½ cup peas
1 pinch dried oregano, or to taste
½ tsp. ground cumin
1 tbsp. red wine vinegar or umeboshi vinegar, to taste
Fresh black pepper, to taste
Garnish: chopped parsley

Preparation:

1. Wash and soak garbanzos for 8 hours. Drain, place in large soup pot, and add 5 cups fresh water or *Vegetable Stock with Herbs* from this Step, and the bay leaf.
2. Bring to boil and then simmer for about 1.5 hours, or pressure cook for 50 minutes (or according to your pressure cooker's timetable). Discard bay leaf.
3. Take out one cup of beans and mash with a potato masher or electric blender and return to pot (or make hummus). Add sea salt and simmer 5 minutes.
4. Meanwhile, heat oil on medium in a skillet. Sauté the onions (optional), garlic (optional), carrot, celery, and celery root for a few minutes. Add to the garbanzos.
5. Bring to a boil, add peas, oregano, and cumin, and simmer till vegetables are soft.
6. Toward the end, add vinegar and a dash of black pepper and stir.
7. Serve garnished with plenty of parsley.

Variations:

- Use two 14.5 ounce cans garbanzo beans, rinsed and drained, for a quick soup.
- Spice it up with 1 tsp. dried basil, 1 tsp. dry mustard, or ¼ tsp. saffron.
- Make a *Sweet Garbanzo Stew:* add 1½ cup diced autumn squash. Omit oregano, cumin, and black pepper and use tahini and sweet chickpeas miso as seasoning instead.

Breakfast or Anytime Dishes

Water Cleanse: Drink a glass of room temperature water first thing in the morning to replenish your liquids. Adding lemon juice will help your acid-alkaline balance.

Plum Vegetable Soup

4 servings

Perk up your appetite by serving small bowls of this soup to start your day. Enjoy it any time as a quick pick-me-up, or serve it before your main meal. For a healing effect, drink this soup about a half hour before your meal.

Ingredients:

4 cups filtered or spring water, or stock
1 cup tofu, finely cubed
2 tsp. wakame flakes, rinsed
1 umeboshi plum, or to taste
Garnish: sliced scallions, and/or finely chopped nori slivers

Preparation:

1. Bring water, tofu, and wakame flakes to a quick boil.
2. Mince or finely chop the umeboshi plum, or use equal amount of umeboshi paste.
3. Reduce heat to low and simmer for 3-5 minutes. Serve with garnish of your choice.

Variations:

1. Use umeboshi vinegar instead of the plum.
2. Add your favorite miso to the broth and adjust the plum content.
3. Add a few sprigs of greens like watercress, bok choy, or Chinese (Napa) cabbage.
4. Use a variety of seasonal vegetables like daikon or shiitake mushrooms.

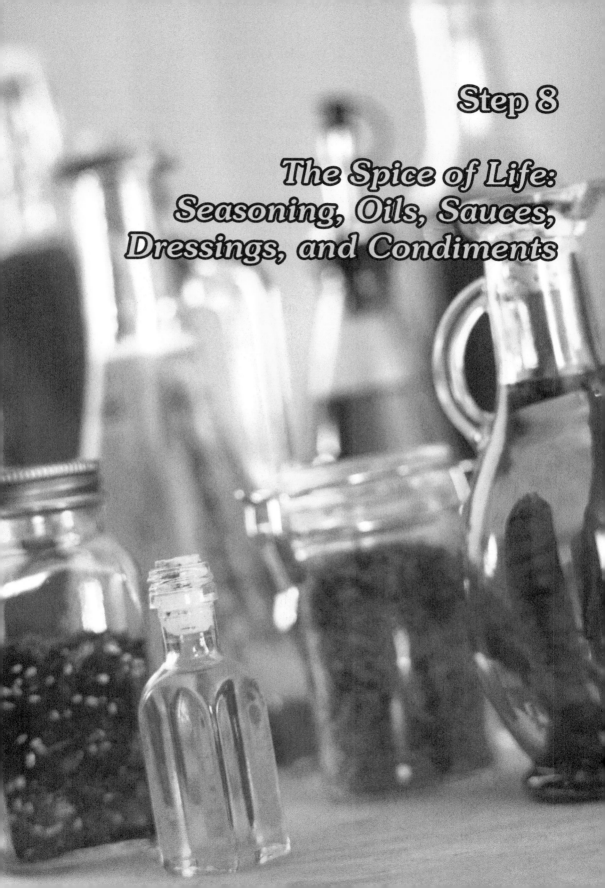

Step 8

**The Spice of Life:
Seasoning, Oils, Sauces,
Dressings, and Condiments**

To bring variety and adventure to the nutritious dishes you make with fresh produce, serve them with healthful oils and tasty condiments, dressings, and sauces. Make your cooking easier by organizing the seasonings in your natural pantry according to the five tastes of sour, bitter, sweet, pungent, and salty. It is definitely worth your experimentation to learn how you can bring any or all of the five tastes to your meals and enhance their nutrient content at the same time.

Some naturally processed dressings and seasonings are available for purchase, so stocking your whole foods pantry is easier than you think. If you wish to entirely avoid condiments that are loaded with sugar, corn syrup, and other undesirable additives, you can create your own during this Step. At a restaurant, if you just ask for oil, sea salt, and lemon when ordering a salad, you can make your own dressing there too.

Condiments, dressings, and sauces are easy to make and can be stored in the refrigerator. A condiment sprinkled over food, like gomasio (a sea salt and crushed sesame mix), or eaten as a side dish, such as a tablespoon of sauerkraut, is all you need to start enjoying their appetite and digestion-stimulating effects.

Seasonings and Condiments According to the Five Tastes

Experiment with all the seasonings and seek out ingredients, condiments, and products that fit into the following five taste classifications. Throughout this book you will find inspirations on how to use them in your recipes. Refer to the *Staples for Your Natural Foods Kitchen* and the *Glossary of Terms* for further ideas.

Sour

Sauerkraut, apple cider vinegar, homemade pickles, brown rice vinegar, umeboshi plums, umeboshi vinegar, lemon and lemon rinds, lime and lime rinds.

Bitter

Tekka condiment, nori, parsley, dandelion, and walnuts.

Sweet

Sweet rice miso, chickpea miso, applesauce, barley malt (contains gluten), brown rice syrup, brown rice malt (contains gluten), mirin, and raisins.

Pungent:

Scallions, watercress, onions, chives, daikon, ginger root, garlic, mustard, black pepper, and horseradish.

Salty

Sea salt, gomasio, wakame powder, barley miso (contains gluten), soy miso, brown rice miso, tamari, soy sauce (contains gluten), and shoyu (contains gluten).

Healthy Considerations for Spices, Herbs, and Salt

Spices and herbs have strong healing properties, so use them with respect, most often sparingly. Salt has a place in every kitchen, if properly used. Every culture has its own traditions—explore what the world has to offer to your kitchen and enhance your food enjoyment.

Sea Salt

Choose natural sea salt instead of regular table salt that has been chemically enhanced. A few sprinkles or a pinch of good quality sea salt enhance the taste of the food by drawing out its flavor, a yin property of salt. Because salt is very yang, you need only small amounts to receive its health benefits of smooth metabolism with steady energy and focused mind. The unrefined minerals in sea salt are essential to the body's ability to make strong blood, bones, teeth, nerves, tissues, and cells.

Spices

Hot spices like chilies are known to stimulate the nervous system and numb the taste buds, so don't overuse them. If you like to add heat to your dishes, you can opt instead for milder spices like ginger, turmeric, coriander, cumin, black pepper, or Ceylon cinnamon that support your health and don't overstimulate your system. Ginger has a special place in macrobiotic cuisine. This pungent, yet sweetly fragrant spice can help to stimulate the appetite and increase circulation. Drunk as a tea, it may ease coughing, lower fever, and reduce pain. Some research suggests that it may benefit the circulatory system by slowing blood clotting.

Herbs

Add fresh, in-season (yin) or dried (yang) herbs to enhance the flavor and nutrient content of your dishes. Note that you will use a greater amount of fresh than dried herbs to achieve the desired effect. Frequently use freshly minced parsley, scallions, chives, basil, mint, or cilantro as garnish or mixed in. Occasionally add fresh or dried thyme, sage, oregano, rosemary, or tarragon to bring a variety of natural tastes and nutrients.

What Kind of Oils to Use in Your Macrobiotic Kitchen

Fats are an essential part of our diet, as they provide the cells with fuel and supply raw material for various chemical, protective, and cushioning functions in the whole body. Fats are also necessary to enable the fat-soluble vitamins A, D, E, and K to be absorbed from food.

There are numerous types of dietary fats and oils. They are all composed primarily of fatty acids—monounsaturated (MUFAs), polyunsaturated (PUFAs), saturated, or trans-unsaturated. Depending on the food source and how they are processed, the fatty acid composition in a given fat or oil will vary.

Most oils from plant sources, such as seeds, beans, fruits, and nuts, have relatively little saturated fat, and are mostly composed of MUFAs and PUFAs. There are some exceptions, such as the tropical palm and coconut oils, which are mostly saturated.

Animal fats are generally higher in saturated fats, but also contain MUFAs and PUFAs. Fish oils are among the few from animal sources that are relatively high in

PUFAs, and are a particularly good source of eicosapentaenoic acid (EPA, i.e., a fatty acid that is twenty ("eicosa") carbon atoms long and has five ("penta") unsaturated bonds—hence, "polyunsaturated"), as well as docosahexaenoic acid (DHA, twenty-two carbon atoms long with six unsaturated bonds). Naturally occurring dietary trans fats are found in small quantities in beef fat, pork fat, and butter.

Hydrogenated oils and synthetic trans fats that are made during food processing are found in many commercial foods.

Emphasize MUFA and PUFA-Rich Oils, Nuts, and Seeds

Scientific research regarding nutritional aspects of oils and fats is constantly evolving. Yet numerous studies have demonstrated that eating foods that are rich in MUFAs and PUFAs can be an important part of a healthy diet and can play a role in lowering the risks of heart disease, obesity, cancer, and type 2 diabetes.[84]

The oils that nourish your body best are those that have been used traditionally, such as MUFA- and PUFA-rich olive oil or sesame oil. Other healthy oils to consider for cooking with higher heat are avocado, grape seed, or rice bran oil. Good oils to use only in raw, uncooked form, as in salad dressings, are hazelnut, hemp, walnut, almond, and flax oils. To reap the most benefits, use cold-pressed and unprocessed oils. You can drizzle them over raw or cooked foods before serving. Store oils, and oil-rich foods such as seeds and nuts, in the refrigerator. This can help prevent oxidation of the PUFAs and prevent the oils from going rancid.

Consume foods such as nuts and seeds that are naturally rich in healthy MUFAs and PUFAs. There are a wide variety of these foods that even in small quantities can add variety and flavor to your meals. Some that are widely available include almonds, hazelnuts, hemp seeds, peanuts, pecans, pine nuts, pistachios, walnuts, cashews, macadamias, and sunflower or pumpkin seeds. Include these in small amounts, raw, sprouted, or occasionally lightly roasted and salted, in your meal planning.

Specifics on MUFA and PUFA and Their Omega 3, 6, and 9 Fatty Acid Content

It is commonly thought that one needs to have an appropriate balance of omega-6, omega-3, as well as omega-9 fatty acids in the diet. All three are necessary for bodily function and health. Unsaturated MUFA-rich oils with their omega-9 nonessential fatty acids have health benefits,[85] and diets rich in these oils have been shown to support immune function. Omega-9 fatty acids are called "nonessential" because our body can make them if there are enough omega-3 and omega-6 essential fatty acids available in the body.

PUFAs are omega-3 and omega-6 essential fatty acids. "Essential" means that these nutrients cannot be synthesized by human metabolism. Animal fats generally contain lower concentrations of omega-3 and omega-6 PUFAs compared to vegetable oils because animals, like humans, are unable to synthesize these fatty acids. Thus, the amounts of PUFAs vary from food to food, with most vegetable oils containing larger amounts than most animal fats.

Most people do not need to worry about getting enough omega-6 fatty acids, as they are abundant in any even moderately healthy diet—soy and corn oil contain plenty of them. Omega-3 fatty acids, on the other hand, may require your conscious attention, as their maximum benefits are obtained by taking care to eat sufficient foods that contain these fatty acids, raw and uncooked. The three major types of omega-3 fatty acids that are found naturally in foods include ALA (alpha-linolenic acid), EPA, and DHA. Substantial amounts of ALA are found in many nut and seed oils. Flaxseed and its oil are particularly rich sources. (See the list under What Kind of Seeds and Nuts to Eat.) The best sources of EPA and DHA, however, are fatty fish such as halibut, mackerel, lake trout, herring, sardines, albacore tuna, and salmon. Your body can make EPA and DHA from ALA, and thus oils rich in ALA can provide a source of omega-3 fatty acids for people who want to avoid fish. However, fish remains the best source of these fatty acids, especially if you do not take supplements.

Adequate intake of omega-3 fatty acids has been demonstrated to have numerous health benefits. They have been shown in studies to help the heart,[86] joints[87], and brain function.[88] As a result, ground seeds and oils rich in omega-3 have become increasingly popular as supplements.

Some Cautions Apply: Even though omega-3 fatty acids (ALA) from flax meal might reduce heart disease mortality, epidemiologic studies also showed an increased risk of prostate cancer in men with a high intake or blood level of ALA.[89] (If you plan to take supplements, please follow the advice of your nutritionist and physician.)

Minimize Saturated Fats and Their Food Sources

Many high-level medical and governmental authorities such as the World Health Organization[90] and the European Food Safety Authority[91] advise that high intake of saturated fatty acids can be risk factor for cardiovascular disease.

Saturated fatty acids are also found in most fats and oils, but the foods that have the largest quantities of saturated fatty acids are usually derived from animal sources. These include dairy foods such as milk, cheese, and ice cream; fats from animal sources such as butter and lard; and red meats such as beef, pork, or lamb. If you use these foods in your macrobiotic kitchen, do so only occasionally, in moderation, and with plenty of vegetables. (See Step 3 for ideas.) Although eggs are not a particularly high source of saturated fatty acids, they contain cholesterol, and may raise your blood cholesterol levels and thus affect your risk of cardiovascular diseases. However, the effects of eggs on blood cholesterol have shown considerable diversity in different individuals. Eggs for one person might be part of a healthy diet but for another increase their cholesterol.[92]

Animal foods are also the only source of cholesterol in the diet, as plants do not synthesize this compound. Eating these foods can raise cholesterol levels, and increase the likelihood of getting heart disease, diabetes, and some cancers, including colon cancer. While these adverse impacts are not due solely to the cholesterol, by minimizing eating these foods, you also minimize most concentrated dietary sources of saturated fats.

Some tropical vegetable oils, such as coconut oil or palm oil, are also high in saturated fatty acids. Coconut oil has shown some health benefits. The long-term health effects of consuming coconut oil on a regular basis are, however, largely not well known. Populations that traditionally consume such oils, such as Pacific Islanders, have also traditionally eaten little red meat, consumed regular fish and seafood and an abundance of fruits and vegetables, and were physically active. When those populations have shifted to more Western diets and lifestyles, this has resulted in rampant obesity, diabetes, and other metabolic disorders.

Avoid Hydrogenated Oils and Foods with Trans Fatty Acids

Synthetically manufactured trans fats are found mostly in vegetable oils that have undergone hydrogenation. As hydrogenation also increases shelf life, these oils are likely to be found in processed foods such as margarines, vegetable shortening, partially hydrogenated vegetable oils, deep-fried fast foods such as doughnuts and French fries that have been prepared in these oils, and many commercially baked goods such as crackers, cookies, and cakes.

Many food producers have reduced or eliminated trans fats from their preparation methods, recognizing their negative health effects, which include increased risks of cardiovascular disease and type 2 diabetes.[93] Yet, check your food labels. If an ingredient lists "hydrogenated" or "partially hydrogenated" vegetable oils, it likely contains trans fats. (Note that trans fat content of less than 0.5 grams per serving does not need to be listed on labels in the US at the time of this publication.)

Pros and Cons for Oils, Seeds, and Nuts

Pros:

- Olive oil can be beneficial for persons with high blood pressure. The polyphenols in this food can help to relax the blood vessels through an increase in nitric oxide production.[94]
- Using fresh extra virgin olive oil in your kitchen might not only have a helpful effect on your cholesterol, but as researchers have discovered, it might have anti-inflammatory effects.
- Using oils such as olive oil that are rich in monounsaturated fats instead of animal fats such as butter that are rich in saturated fats is an easy way to improve the healthfulness of your food choices.[95]
- Some vegetable oils, such as sesame oil or flaxseed oil, contain powerful antioxidants called lignans, which may also be anti-carcinogenic. They may also contain phytosterols, which are believed to reduce blood levels of cholesterol, enhance the immune response, and decrease risk of certain cancers when present in the diet in sufficient amounts.
- According to one study,[96] sesame seeds have one of the highest levels of total phytosterol (400-413 mg per 100 grams/3.5 ounces). Among the seeds and nuts typically consumed as snack foods, pistachios and sunflower seeds were richest in phytosterols (270-289 mg/100 g, followed by pumpkin seeds, 265 mg/100 g).
- It is not necessary to avoid healthy fats and oils. Many studies have shown that people who follow a Mediterranean-type diet are less likely to develop heart disease. The Mediterranean diet is not necessarily low in oils, and in some places, including those countries that have traditionally had low rates of heart disease such as Greece or Southern Italy; olive oil is enjoyed as a part of traditional cuisine. The Mediterranean diet is associated with good health for a number of reasons, and it includes not only olive oil and olives, but also whole grains, fresh fruits and vegetables, seeds and nuts, fish, and garlic, as well as moderate wine consumption.

Cons:

- Fats and oils contain the most calories for a given quantity of any food, and a diet with unhealthy high fat content may also be high in calories, with associated risk of weight gain. Gaining excess weight has numerous health consequences. It is a major contributor to high blood pressure, cardiovascular disease, risk of some cancers and diabetes, and other health issues. So, avoiding unhealthy fatty and oily foods, as well as sugar-containing foods, will help you maintain a healthy body weight.
- To reduce the risk of heart disease, avoid hydrogenated trans fatty acids; there is no good reason to eat foods that contain them.

What Kinds of Seeds and Nuts to Eat

Nuts and seeds like almonds, hazelnuts, hemp, peanuts, pecans, pine nuts, pistachios, walnuts, sunflower seeds, flaxseeds, and pumpkin seeds are just some of the many foods that can be enjoyed as part of a healthful diet. But because the oils in these nuts and seeds are high in polyunsaturated fatty acids, they are prone to rancidity and oxidation when exposed to heat, and may thus lose the benefits of their omega-3 essence. While they may be enjoyed roasted and cooked in various dishes, they can also be eaten in uncooked form to maximize the health benefits of the oils. You can eat them raw or sprouted as snacks, or soak and grind them to make your own nut milks. Add them as a garnish on salads, grains, or beans, but don't use them in highly salted or sugared forms.

As nuts and seeds are high in calories and are dense foods, it is difficult to consume large quantities at any one time. But eating a handful a day, perhaps 1.5 ounces, (42.5 grams), or using them as a garnish or flavoring agent, is a delicious way to incorporate small amounts into your diet. Other food sources that have oils in only small amounts, but are rich in omega-3 essential fatty acids, can also be eaten daily. Examples include mustard seeds, green leafy vegetables, sea vegetables, spirulina, and whole grains.

Sesame seeds are one of the oldest cultivated plants in the world. Throughout the ages, from Babylon and Assyria to India, China, and Japan, sesame oil has been highly prized for cooking, in sesame cakes, as medicine, for ceremonial purification, and as a base for perfumes and inks. Sesame grows in most tropical, subtropical, and southern temperate areas of the world. Sesame seeds are very tiny (yang) and come in a variety of colors, from cream-white to charcoal-black. You will love their nutty flavor in cooking (although high heat damages their healthful polyunsaturated fats). You can use them daily as sesame sea salt (gomasio), a condiment to shake over rice and other cooked grains, bean dishes, and salads. From sesame teas to ginger-sesame oil, rice syrup-sweetened sesame treats, and rice crackers, sesame seeds are easy to add to many dishes. Sesame seeds also come ground as tahini paste (raw or toasted) and can be used in various recipes, such as hummus or sauces.

Aspects of Cooking with Oil

Choose organic, expeller-pressed unrefined oils. These processes do not use heat or solvents to extract the oils from nuts, fruits, or seeds, and thus these oils retain most of their nutrients. Expeller and cold pressing also minimize the oxidation of these unsaturated fatty acids, which preserves their taste.

Preserving the nutrients of oil during cooking requires some attention. All oils have different smoking points, so check with the label to match your desired cooking style. For health or taste reasons, you can sauté your food with a few tablespoons of water instead of oil, adding the optional oil when food is still warm before serving. When you cook with water, the taste opens up and is released in the steam.

Oils for Medium and Low Heat Cooking

For daily cooking (medium and low heat), use light expeller-pressed extra virgin olive oil or unrefined light sesame oil. Both will enhance the flavors of food. Sesame oil, with its high PUFA and MUFA content, is also rich in the natural antioxidants *sesamin* and *sesamol*, and is therefore not prone to oxidation. Light sesame oil has a mild, nutty flavor and can be used either raw or in cooking on medium heat. Olive oil and olives have been used for thousands of years, and their oils are still a favorite in many cuisines. For cooking (medium and low heat), use light expeller-pressed extra virgin olive oil.

It is best to heat these oils on low to medium flame, between 130 and 139° F (90–95° C). Use high-quality stainless steel or cast iron cookware to ensure even heat. Make sure the oil doesn't start smoking. If it does, you may want to discard it and start again. Test the heat level with a piece of the food that you are going to cook (onion works fine), and when the oil starts to sizzle, add the rest of the food you want to sauté, resulting in a natural cooling down to the correct heat level. This way, the food will be evenly heated and the nutrients and taste captured, enhanced, and concentrated.

Oils for High-Heat Cooking

For high heat stir-fries, or the occasional deep-frying or tempura making, choose oils with a higher smoking point, such as rice bran oil, which has a smoking point of about 415° F (213° C). This property of rice bran oil is the reason it is often used for Japanese tempura. With its high MUFA and vitamin E content, rice bran oil may also benefit health by providing antioxidants and lowering blood pressure. Grapeseed oil, with its high smoke point of 485° F (252° C) and high vitamin E content, is a daily favorite of European chefs as a healthy choice for high-heat cooking, as well as in condiments or salad dressings. Another choice that is becoming increasingly popular is unrefined virgin avocado oil, with a smoking point between 375-400° F (=190-204° C).

Using Oils Raw, Without Cooking

Oils like flaxseed that contain lignans, and nut oils like hemp, walnut, or hazelnut, provide omega-3 and omega-6 essential fatty acids (the ones the body cannot make). If you choose these oils, do not heat them if you wish to receive their benefits. Buy these oils refrigerated and store them cold, as they get rancid easily. Use only about one teaspoon per day, in salad dressings or poured over cereals or pasta dishes, and adjust your intake of cooked oils accordingly.

Choose cold-pressed extra virgin olive oil, which comes from the first pressing of the olives. "Cold-pressed" means that no heat was used to extract the extra virgin olive oil, making this an ideal flavorful oil to use cold, as in salad dressings.

Dark sesame oil has an intense flavor from the roasting of the sesame seeds prior to extracting the oil. Use it mostly to flavor already cooked dishes.

Tips for Storing Oils

Keep your oils in the refrigerator to prevent them from getting rancid. Some oils, like olive and coconut oil, will solidify when stored in the refrigerator, yet they will return to liquid when warmed to room temperature. You can store them in wide-mouth containers so you can scoop them out like butter, using only what you need for that meal's preparation, instead of bringing the whole bottle to room temperature. Or you can pour a week's supply of your favorite cooking oil into a smaller bottle to have handy on the kitchen shelf.

Seasonal and Yin-Yang Tidbits for Oils

The olive, a fruit, is yin compared to sesame, a seed, which is more yang. To achieve balance when using oils, choose olive oil (yin) more in the summer (yang) and sesame oil (yang) more in the winter (yin). Choose heated oils (yang) for cooking more in the winter (yin) and cold oils (yin) more in the summer (yang).

Recipes for The Spice of Life: Seasoning, Oils, Sauces, Dressings, and Condiments

Sesame Sea Salt Table Condiment

Adjustable sprinkle servings

This combination of sesame seeds that are rich in protein, calcium, iron, and B vitamins with sea salt, a great source of trace minerals, calcium, iron, potassium, manganese, magnesium, iodine, and zinc, is a powerful condiment we call *gomasio*. You need only sprinkles to reap a range of health benefits. The aromas that fill your kitchen are so wonderful that you won't want to miss making your own gomasio . . . often.

Ingredients:

6 tbsp. whole brown sesame seeds
1 tsp. sea salt
Suribachi or seed and nut-dedicated coffee grinder

Preparation:

1. Wash sesame seeds and drain them in a strainer. Place the strainer on a dry towel to absorb most of the liquid.
2. Roast sea salt for a few minutes in a stainless steel skillet until it is shiny.
3. Grind sea salt in suribachi or coffee grinder to a fine powder.
4. Place sesame seeds in a dry skillet and roast on a low-medium flame, stirring constantly with a wooden spoon and shaking the skillet from time to time.
5. When the seeds give off a nutty fragrance, become light golden brown, and begin popping, crush one between your fingers. If it crushes easily, the seeds are done.
6. Place the seeds in the suribachi containing the ground sea salt, and slowly grind with an even, circular motion until each seed is half-crushed. If using a coffee grinder, grind well, but not so much that they become sesame butter.
7. Store gomasio in a covered glass jar in a cool place. It will keep for about one week in refrigerator.
8. Serve sprinkles over grain dishes, salads, and vegetables.

Variations:

*   Use less sea salt depending on your condition and taste.
*   Omit the sea salt and grind the seeds with roasted wakame sea vegetable.
*   Use black sesame seeds—they contain less oil then the brown seeds, or use a mix of both. Whole brown or black sesame seeds are preferable to white ones.

Avocado and Basil Dip

4 to 5 servings

Use this dressing as a dip for vegetables. Avocados contain oleic acid, a monounsaturated fat that may help lower cholesterol. Avocados are a good source of potassium, a mineral that helps regulate blood pressure. Tofu provides easily absorbable protein.

Ingredients:
4 ounces soft tofu
Water/tamari mixture (50/50), enough to cover tofu
7 basil leaves, washed
2 avocados
1 lemon, juice and zest
1/8 tsp. sea salt
Filtered water or extra virgin olive oil, to taste
Tamari to reseason (optional)

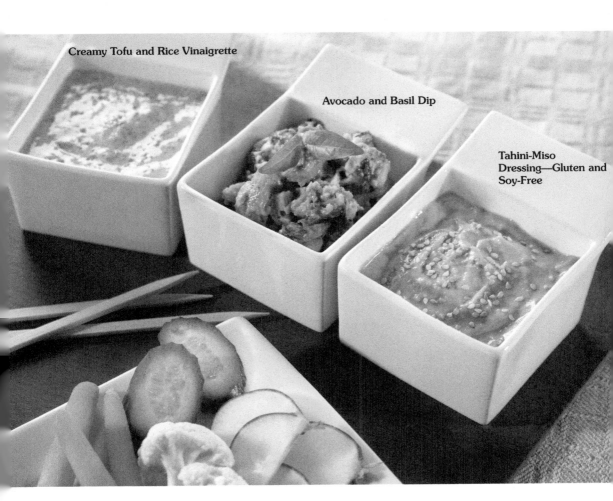

Creamy Tofu and Rice Vinaigrette

Avocado and Basil Dip

Tahini-Miso Dressing—Gluten and Soy-Free

Preparation:
1. Cube the tofu and boil it in the water/tamari mixture for 5 minutes. Remove, drain, and set aside.
2. Wash and finely cut the basil.
3. Slice avocado in half, remove the seed, and scoop out the soft green avocado flesh.
4. Combine the avocado flesh, tofu, basil, lemon juice and zest, and sea salt in a blender or food processor. Purée until smooth while adding drizzles of water or oil to reach a smooth consistency. Reseason with tamari if needed.
5. Serve at room temperature. Eat as a dip with raw or slightly steamed vegetables.
6. Store in refrigerator.

Variations:
- Mix into the dip a variety of finely chopped raw or steamed vegetables like celery or carrots for a different texture and taste.
- Use avocado oil instead of olive oil.
- Serve over cooked grain, or mix with a noodle dish.

Creamy Tofu and Rice Vinaigrette

(included in Avocado Basil Dressing photo, p. 157)

4–6 servings

Use this delicious vinaigrette on salads or over steamed vegetables, noodles, or sea vegetable dishes.

Ingredients:
1–2 cups soft tofu
2 cups filtered or spring water
1 tbsp. tamari, or to taste
1 tbsp. brown rice vinegar
1 tsp. extra virgin olive oil or flax oil with lignans
Turmeric, to taste

Preparation:
1. Cut the tofu into large pieces and boil in water/tamari mix for 5 minutes.
2. Remove and drain the excess water/tamari liquid from the tofu. Set liquid aside.
3. Blend, or food-process tofu, brown rice vinegar, oil, and turmeric until smooth.
4. If needed, add some of the set aside water/tamari mixture for a smoother texture.
5. Store in a cool place for up to 5 days.
6. Add a good amount of this vinaigrette to your dishes, or serve as a dip with vegetables.

Variations:
- Simmer the tofu in a water/miso mixture for 5 minutes.
- Blend in ginger juice, herbs such as basil or chives, or a small piece of avocado.

Vegan Mock Bacon Condiment

Adjustable servings (Scrambled Tofu from step 3, p. 76, is included in this photo)

This condiment works best with purchased *takuan* daikon pickles. It goes well with many grain dishes, or use it in the morning to replace your bacon—it tastes good with the breakfast recipes from this book, or serve it with the *Scrambled Tofu* dish from Step 3, as seen in the photo.

Ingredients:

2 tbsp. light sesame oil
Takuan daikon pickles, wiped and sliced
Tamari, to taste; Few drops filtered or spring water

Preparation:

1. Heat oil in a skillet, add the takuan pickle slices, and brown them on both sides.
2. Season with tamari, add a few drops of water, cover, and simmer on low a minute or two.

Variations:

- Use the Sea Salt-Pressed Red Radishes from Step 5 instead of purchasing the takuan pickle.

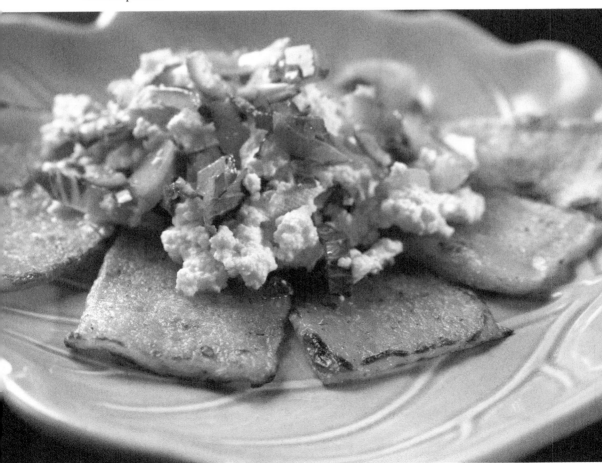

Gabriele's Favorite Dressing

4 servings

Drizzle this dressing over raw salad, cooked green leafy vegetables, or steamed root and round vegetables. Make a large batch and store in the refrigerator to have it always on hand.

Ingredients:

9 tbsp. filtered or spring water
1 tbsp. lemon juice or umeboshi, rice, or balsamic vinegar
Pinches sea salt or herbal salt, to taste
1–2 tbsp. extra virgin olive oil
1 tbsp. chopped scallions or parsley
1 tbsp. tamari (optional)
3 cloves garlic, minced and lightly sautéed in oil (optional)
¼ tsp. basil minced (optional)
Garnish: dill, several sprigs

Preparation:

1. Whisk ingredients together, adjusting the water/vinegar/oil ratio to your liking to find out your favorite combinations.
2. Whisk in other optional ingredients or shake them into the mix in a closed container.
3. Drizzle over cooked greens or a raw salad and garnish with dill.
4. Store leftover dressing in a closed glass container in the refrigerator for about 4 days.

Variations:

• Add mustard or soymilk to change the taste and color.
• Add orange juice and orange slices, or avocado pieces, to taste.

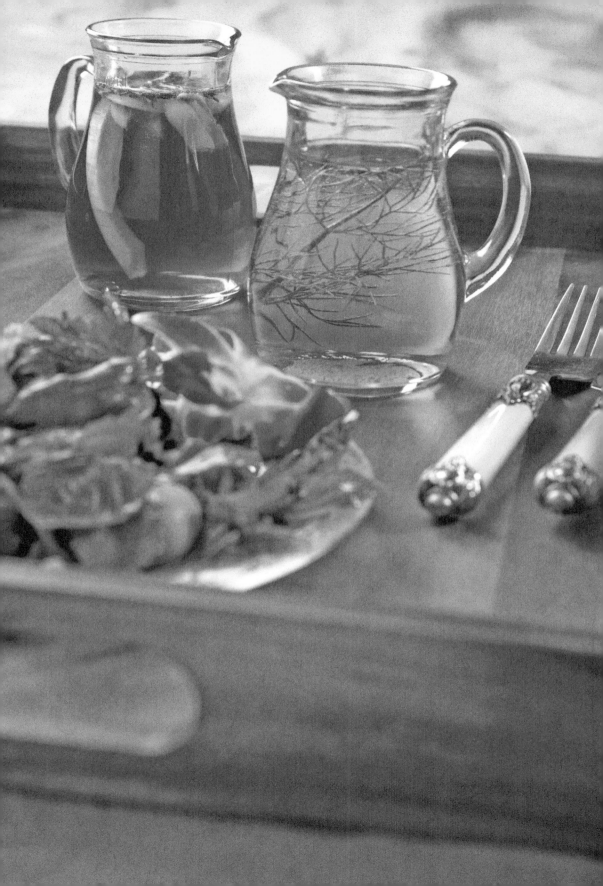

Dairy and Egg-Free Vegan Mayonnaise

4 servings

This is a great gluten-, dairy-, and egg-free vegan mayonnaise to have on hand, as it goes well with many dishes. For a delicious coleslaw effect, mix it with shredded cabbage and carrots and let marinate for one hour before serving. It is the perfect spread for a sandwich. (See Step 1 to refresh your knowledge about dairy foods.)

Ingredients:

1 cup tofu, regular or silken, drained
2 tsp. apple cider vinegar
2 tsp. Dijon mustard
2 tsp. maple syrup
1 tbsp. extra virgin olive oil
1 tsp. herbal blend of your choice
Filtered or spring water, as needed

Preparation:

1. Combine all ingredients in an electric blender and mix to a thick but creamy consistency.
2. Adjust seasoning to taste. If needed, add some water and continue mixing.
3. Keeps in the refrigerator for about 2 days.
4. Variations:
5. Use different vinegars like umeboshi or brown rice.
6. Use different sweeteners like gluten-free brown rice syrup, or omit all sweeteners.
7. Add turmeric for added nutrients and color.

Variations:

- Use different vinegars like umeboshi or brown rice.
- Use different sweeteners like gluten-free brown rice syrup, or omit all sweeteners.
- Add turmeric for added nutrients and color.

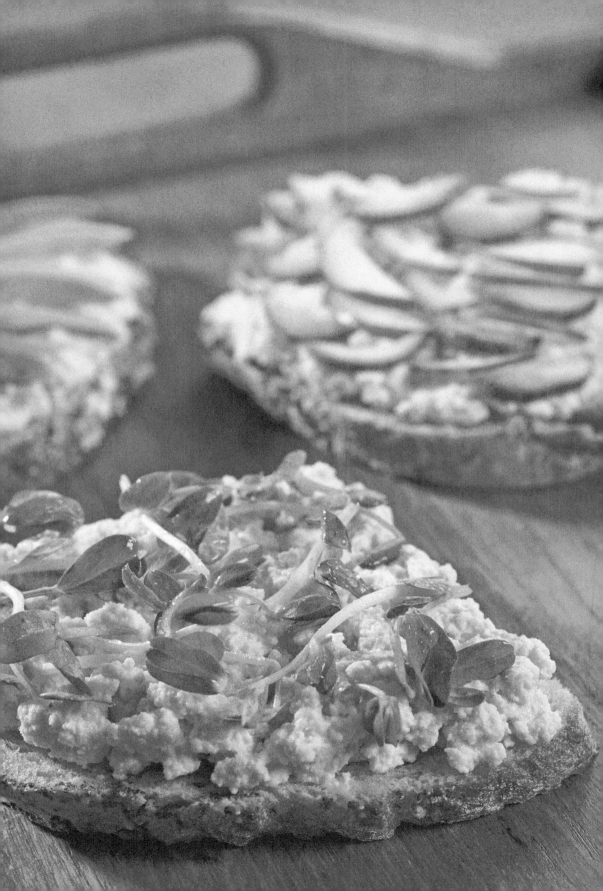

Tahini-Miso Dressing—Gluten and Soy-Free

(included in Avocado Basil Dressing photo, p. 157)

1–2 servings

To help green leafy vegetables become a favorite on your family's table, top them with a spoonful of this rich-tasting dressing. It will convince even the pickiest eater to try a bite (or two or three). Or it can also be served as a dip with vegetables.

Ingredients:

2 tbsp. chickpea miso
1 tbsp. tahini sesame butter
½ tsp. tamari
½ tsp. lemon juice
Filtered or spring water as needed
Garnish: toasted sesame seeds

Preparation:

1. Combine miso, tahini, tamari, and lemon juice in a suribachi or electric blender. Or use a bowl to mix with fork.
2. Add water gradually and continue mixing till smooth and creamy to achieve your desired consistency.
3. Spoon this dressing over your favorite steamed greens. If needed, squeeze cooked greens before adding the dressing to remove excess water.

Variations:

- Add chopped herbs like basil, parsley, and chives.
- Add umeboshi paste, umeboshi vinegar, or grated daikon, and omit the tamari.
- Add tofu, pressed for 5 minutes and then steamed or blanched.
- Use fresh sesame seeds instead of tahini: wash and drip-dry the sesame seeds in a strainer, then toast in a skillet till slightly browned. Grind them in a suribachi or a coffee grinder. Add water until you have the desired consistency.
- For a stronger taste, use gluten and soybean-free adzuki bean miso.

Mushroom-Onion Sauce with Tamari and Ginger

(photo of this sauce is included in Step 4, p.92, Mashed Potato Style Parsnips,

3–4 servings

This sauce is delicious served over grain dishes, especially the millet dish from Step 2, Whole Grains: Beyond Processed Foods, or added to a sandwich, or poured over steamed vegetables or noodles.

Ingredients:
2 cups onions, finely sliced
1 tsp. light sesame oil
2 cups button mushrooms, cleaned and sliced
1 tbsp. tamari, or to taste
Grated ginger or ginger juice, to taste
1–2 cups filtered or spring water
≈ 1 tbsp. arrowroot or kuzu, diluted with 2 tbsp. cold water
Pinch sea salt
Garnish: minced scallions or parsley, or a mix of both

Preparation:
1. Sauté the onions in sesame oil, first on medium, then on low heat until browned.
2. Repeat the above step with mushrooms. Add tamari and ginger to taste.
3. Add water, bring to a quick boil, cover the pan, and simmer on low heat for about 10 minutes.
4. Toward the end, use diluted arrowroot or kuzu to thicken any leftover water.
5. If needed, add more water for a nice sauce. Stir until it thickens.
6. Add a pinch of sea salt, stir, and serve hot, garnished with scallions or parsley.

Variations:
- Instead of tamari, use your favorite herb or spice mixture.
- Add garlic to the mix and omit ginger. Garnish with cilantro or Italian parsley.

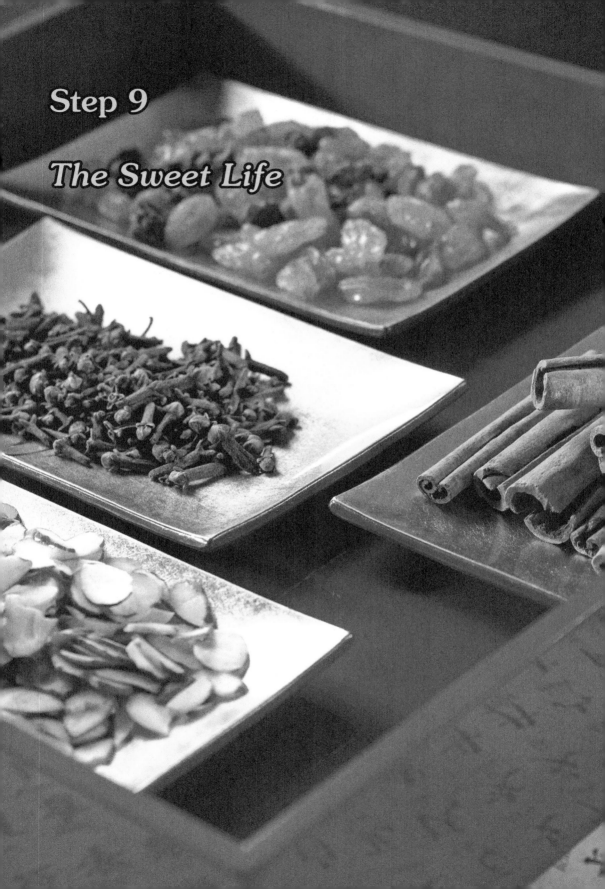

Step 9

The Sweet Life

Sugary treats . . . *mmm*. You can find sweetness in obvious places—candy bars, ice cream, cookies or cakes, soft drinks—and less obvious ones. Sugar is added to most processed, packaged, and canned foods, from sodas to pickles, ketchup, and peanut butter. Many restaurants add sugar to their dishes to make them tastier. During this Step, you will learn to recognize, minimize, and avoid refined, simple sugars and artificial sweeteners. Enjoy the benefits and uses of natural complex sweeteners and sweet tasting vegetables in your kitchen and easy ways to prepare your own delicious desserts.

The Many Names of Refined, Simple, and Chemical Sugars

In the last 500 years, since the first sugar refinery was built, sugar consumption has increased from rare use as a luxury item to an estimated 150 pounds of sugar per year per person in the US. The health implications as well as the environmental impact of sugar production are huge. Besides white sugar (sucrose) from sugarcane, a tropical food, there are many varieties of highly refined and nutrient-devoid sugars added to packaged foods.[97] Here are some of the names so you can avoid them by reading the ingredient lists: confectioners' sugar/powdered sugar, corn syrup, dextrose, high-fructose corn syrup (HFCS), fructose, raw sugar, brown sugar, rapadura, Sucanat, date sugar, xylitol... and the list goes on.[98] Some of these products might even contain gluten or be manufactured with gluten-containing products.

Other forms of simple sugars that are claimed to be better, like agave syrup, coconut sugar, evaporated cane juice, or stevia, have found their way into modern lifestyle products as a replacement for white sugar. Some are also found in gluten-free packaged foods, yet are still sugars, and not necessarily healthy.

Chemical or artificial sweeteners like aspartame, saccharin, sucralose, acesulfame K, neotame, and cyclamate (which is not approved in the United States but is approved for use in other countries) have skyrocketed in use as an alternative to sugar. This is because many people are trying to reduce sugar and calories in the effort to manage their health or lose weight. However, research suggests that chemical sweeteners may be associated with *increased* weight as well as cancer and neurological issues, especially in the case of aspartame.[99] [100] [101]

The sugar content of most packaged foods can be easily understood by converting the grams on the label—4 grams of sugar equals one teaspoon. A small container of blueberry yogurt, for instance, contains 34-40 grams of sugar, or about ten teaspoons. The label words *sugar-free*, *reduced sugar,* or *no added sugar*s do not necessarily mean that there are no sugars at all in a product.

The Unfavorable Effects of Simple and Refined Sugars on Your Body

Refined and simple sugars provide quick energy, but only for a brief time after the rapid raising of the blood sugar level. After that quick rise, the body rapidly releases a rush of insulin, which swiftly lowers the blood sugar and causes a significant drop in energy and endurance. Insulin works to lower blood sugar by pushing it into the body cells, and that is why weight gain happens if this process is repeated often.

When simple or refined sugars enter the stomach, since they are strongly alkaloid the stomach secretes unusual amounts of acid in order to make balance, which, if repeated over a long enough period, can cause eventual ulceration on the stomach wall.

The blood normally maintains a weak alkaline condition, and when strongly alkaline refined sugar is introduced, what is known as an "acid reaction" takes place, causing the bloodstream to become overly acidic. To compensate for this, the internal supply of minerals is mobilized so as to restore a normal balance. The minerals in your daily food and in your normal body reserve are sufficient to meet this situation if it arises now and then. However, if you are eating refined and simple sugars every day, this supply is not sufficient, and you must depend on minerals stored deep within the body, particularly the calcium in your bones and teeth. If this continues for a long enough period, the depletion of calcium from the bones and teeth results in their eventual decay and general weakening.[102]

If you are constantly craving sugary treats, it is important to understand that sugar may play a role in addictive behavior. While it is not addictive in the conventional sense, the more you eat it, the more you want to have foods that are made with refined sugars. William Dufty[103] already pointed this out: "Like heroin, cocaine, and caffeine, sugar is an addictive, destructive drug, yet we consume it daily in everything from cigarettes to bread." A *Journal of Nutrition* article[104] presented information from a number of studies that show that sugar affects brain chemistry in a manner similar to dopamine and may lead to addictive behavior. It also showed that sugar bingeing can cause withdrawal symptoms and cravings comparable to the effects of drug abuse.

Make an experiment and see for yourself. Will you experience any withdrawal symptoms? Leave all sugars out of your diet for several weeks and see how this makes you feel. Do you have a headache? Are you craving it more? After you have abstained from eating any sugar for one month, eat a sugary treat and note your reaction.

The Healthy Effects of Complex Sugars on Your Body

In the normal digestive process, complex sugars that contain fiber, minerals, vitamins, and proteins are first decomposed by the enzymes in the saliva in the mouth, further broken down in the stomach, and then completely digested in the duodenum and intestines. This provides an even energy flow in the body.

In your macrobiotic and natural foods kitchen, choose complex carbohydrate foods like grains, beans, and root and round vegetables. The sugars in these foods are complex sugars such as starch, and when you eat them whole and unprocessed, they also contain dietary fiber. This results in the absorption of their complex sugars in a slow and constant way. They don't spike your blood glucose level and then drop it quickly as with simple sugars added to foods, and so they provide a constant energy supply for your body.

As there is a difference between how the body digests and assimilates simple, refined, and artificial sugars versus complex sugars in food—the former causing disease, with the latter restoring vitality—it is only common sense to reduce processed sugars and foods and increase whole grains, beans, fruits, and vegetables.

Enjoy Your Sweet Life without Added Sugars

Don't go right away for the most accessible sweet treats. You can satisfy your sweet tooth by making delicious dishes with foods like cabbage, onion, winter squashes, fresh corn, chestnuts, or carrots, specially prepared to emphasize their sweet notes. These sweet-tasting vegetables provide health benefits, while refined, simple, and chemical sugary foods have been scientifically shown to cause health challenges. The more you eat these vegetables, the less you will crave the white sugary sweetened stuff. See Step 4 for sweet-tasting vegetable recipes and Step 10 for healthy drinks to immediately satisfy your sugar cravings.

Option: Obtain a sweet taste through eating complex carbohydrate vegetables: Cabbage, Squash, Onions, Parsnips, and Carrots

You will also experience a naturally sweet taste when you chew your whole complex carbohydrate grain dishes thoroughly. This is because the digestive enzymes in your saliva will break down the complex carbohydrates into simpler sugars. Alternate grains according to season and needs, and enjoy a wide variety of brown rice, millet, buckwheat, teff, or quinoa dishes. Refer to Step 3 for recipes.

Yin-Yang Tidbits for Sugars

When you begin to serve macrobiotic yin-yang balanced meals where whole grains are served with a variety of beans, vegetables, greens, soups, and fermented food dishes, you might not beat the sugar cravings immediately. But when you eat these foods regularly, sugar cravings will decrease. These whole and natural foods are rich in complex sugars and taste delicious. When you are eating more vegetable foods (yin) and minimizing or avoiding heavy consumption of salty animal foods (very yang), you will also notice that your cravings for intense sweet sugary tastes will decrease.

Extreme sugar and sweet cravings (very yin) with mood swings and afternoon tiredness could soon be things of the past when paying attention to a quality, more yin-yang balanced lifestyle with whole foods on a daily basis. Better health and a slimmer waist will be the benefits as you embrace this journey of change in your relationship to sugary food.[105]

Natural Complex Sweeteners in Your Kitchen

To add a sweet taste to desserts or beverages, use natural sweeteners in minimal amounts that your body absorbs like normal food. In cooking or in beverages, use natural complex grain sweeteners, natural maple syrup, fresh seasonal or dried fruits, and unsweetened local fruit juices. They have a milder impact on the body than the simple and white sugars in candy bars, doughnuts, or other processed sweet foods.[106]

Even with complex whole foods natural sweeteners, avoid getting into the habit of using them on a daily basis. Learn how to enjoy foods and beverages without sweeteners, and use them only on occasion and in small amounts. Your taste buds will adjust, and you will be able to enjoy and experience the natural flavors of the foods you are eating. Implement all the five flavors—spicy, pungent, bitter, salty, and sweet—in small amounts into your cooking style to provide more taste satisfaction and minimize extreme cravings.

Whole Grain Barley Malt

Barley malt is made from the soaking, sprouting, mashing, cooking, and roasting of barley, a process that capitalizes on the naturally present enzymes. The final product is more of a whole food than many other sweeteners. Barley malt can come in the form of powder or syrup.

Gluten Advice: barley malt contains gluten.

Brown Rice Malt

Has been used in the East for hundreds of years as a sweetener. It contains roughly 30% soluble complex carbohydrate, 45% maltose and other short-chain carbohydrates, 3 to 4% glucose, and 20% water. Glucose, like all the other simple carbohydrates, is absorbed quickly into the blood. The same is largely true for the maltose and short-chain carbohydrates, which consist of two, three, or a handful of glucose compounds strung together, although they can take a bit longer to be digested and absorbed. Brown rice malt is made from brown rice that has been ground and cooked with sprouted barley, and it has also been fermented with natural enzymes from barley malt. Brown rice malt tastes a bit like sweet butterscotch, and is quite delicious. To substitute brown rice malt for sugar in your recipes, use about 50% more brown rice malt syrup than the recipe amount of white sugar, and reduce the amount of other liquids. Brown rice malt syrup has a slightly yang character and digests slowly.

Gluten Advice: barley enzymes and barley malt contain gluten.

Brown Rice Syrup

Also known as "yinnie syrup." It is made from brown rice that has been ground and cooked, and traditionally contains fewer or no naturally fermented barley enzymes. Compared to rice malt syrup, it is lighter colored, more liquid, more yin, and more quickly digested. Newer methods that use a fungal enzyme make brown rice syrup that is gluten free. Check with your source and the ingredient list to see how the rice syrup was made.

Gluten Advice: The enzymes are the key to whether the brown rice syrup is gluten free. When barley enzymes are used to make brown rice syrup, the product is not gluten free.

Amazake

Amazake is a delicious dairy-free sweet drink and natural sweetener made with 100% whole grain brown rice, millet, or other grain. The cultured rice *koji*, *Aspergillus oryzae* (also used to produce tamari and miso), is added to cooked and cooled whole grain. The fermentation that soon occurs causes the enzymes to break down the carbohydrates into complex sugars. As the mixture incubates, the natural sweetness develops, creating a nectar-like beverage. Use it in desserts and as a sweet drink.

Maple Syrup

Maple syrup is harvested from northern climate maple trees, and is a traditional Native American sweetener. One hundred percent pure maple syrup is made from boiled-down maple tree sap and contains many minerals. It adds a pleasant flavor to foods and is great to use in baking instead of white sugar. You can get it as maple sugar, which is about twice as sweet as white sugar but much less refined. It has a more yin note than the whole grain sweeteners and is quickly absorbed into the blood stream. Use it sparingly.

Honey

We don't recommend using honey, as it is sweeter than sugar, and it will spike your blood sugar. When using for its healing properties or as a remedy in certain cases, use it raw or slightly warmed so it will not lose its proclaimed powers. Honey is not a plant-based sweetener.

Fruits in Your Macrobiotic Kitchen

Fruits are wonderful and a delight to eat when in season. Because fruit digests quickly, it provides a quick supply of energy. However, be aware of the balance aspects. When you are eating too many fruits or drinking too much fruit juice in relation to other foods, the body has to deal with excess sugars and liquids.

Glycemic Index and Glycemic Load

Quality and quantity are important considerations in your macrobiotic kitchen. Each food you eat has a different effect on your blood sugar level. Some foods make blood sugar levels rise quickly, and others don't. The glycemic index (GI) provides a measure of how quickly a food can raise blood sugar levels. The glycemic load (GL) takes both the quality and the quantity of the carbohydrate into account. A whole watermelon, for instance, has a glycemic index of 72. This means that it is less likely to cause a rise in blood sugar than the same amount of a reference food, usually table sugar or white bread, which has a glycemic index of 100. Judging from the glycemic index alone, a watermelon would not be safe to eat. However, one serving of 120 grams yields a glycemic load of roughly 4, and therefore would not cause any problems. Consider your health: to keep your sugar levels low, eat only small amounts of seasonal fruits. For some conditions, don't eat them every day, or don't consume fruits at all.

Yin and Yang Tidbits for Fruits

Generally, fruits have yin energy in comparison to vegetables. Fruits cool and refresh you and thus bring balance to your body when you eat them during hotter weather (yang), or when you feel anxious, or your energy feels otherwise contracted (yang). Eating lots of fruits (yin) in the colder winter months (yin), or when you have a yin condition like feeling spacey, can produce an imbalance.

Your immediate locality has the most yang energy for you, and eating the fruits that grow in season in your vicinity (yang) will help to keep your energy balanced, whereas eating fruits from afar (yin) will make balance difficult. In this day and age, when foods are transported from all over the world and available in any season, knowing when and what kind of fruits to eat can be a challenge. The best guide for what kinds of fruits to eat, and when, is to choose locally grown fruits that are in season.

If you live in a four-season climate, for example, eat fruits (yin) from faraway tropical climates (yin) only in very hot (yang) weather that is similar to the weather where the fruit is grown if you want to maintain balance. Pineapples, bananas, oranges, mangoes, figs, dates, kiwi, or coconut are best eaten when you live in or visit a tropical region or on social occasions, or during hot weather. Instead, eat traditionally grown tree fruits like apples, apricots, cherries, grapes, peaches, pears, plums, tangerines, raisins, and currants, or fruits that grow seasonally close to the ground like blueberries, blackberries, cantaloupe, honeydew melon, raspberries, strawberries, and watermelon.

You can transform the energy of raw fruits (yin) by adding yang energy through heat, cooking, dehydration, or sea salt. Making a dessert using these methods allows you to enjoy eating fruits during the cold season without bringing the body out of balance (if done in moderation). Adding a sprinkle of sea salt to either cooked or raw fruits concentrates their sweet flavor and makes them more digestible.

Pros and Cons for the Sweet Life

Pros:

- Fruits have nutritional value and should be part of a yin and yang balanced lifestyle. Eating in season like half an apple, a small slice of melon, or a few grapes or strawberries is a quick way to add flavor and nutrit--ion. Apple skins contain antioxidants as well as flavonoids that enhance the activity of vitamin C and thereby help to lower the risk of heart attack, stroke, and colon cancer. Strawberries have among the highest antioxidant levels of major fruits and protect the body from cancer-causing, blood vessel-clogging free radicals. Watermelons are composed of 92% water and contain vitamin C; potassium; glutathione, which is known to boost the immune system; and lycopene, which has found a place as a cancer-fighting antioxidant.
- Some fruits have cosmetic properties. Strawberries, for example, have the power to brighten your teeth! They contain a lot of malic acid, a tooth-whitening agent.

  Recipe: Use 1 strawberry and ½ teaspoon of baking soda. Crush the strawberry to a pulp; mix it with the baking soda until blended. Use a soft toothbrush to spread the mixture onto your teeth. Leave it on for 5 minutes, and then brush thoroughly with toothpaste to remove the berry-baking soda mix. Rinse. Floss to remove remaining tiny strawberry seeds.

Cons:

- Besides being an obvious cause of tooth decay, the overconsumption of simple sugars can be related to many different health risks: obesity, hypoglycemia, weakened eyesight, suppressed immune system, depression, addictions, diabetes, hypertension[107], and headaches, including migraines.
- Diets high in refined starch and refined sugar may increase the risk of stomach and bowel cancer.[108] Other studies and articles cited earlier in this Step suggest further ill effects from eating sugar.[109]

- Eating large amounts of fruits can cause high blood pressure, at first, and then can weaken the heart to create low blood pressure.
- If you eat excess fruit, either local or tropical, or drink fruit juices, the fruit sugars can cause fatigue and mood or energy swings.
- All foods, especially fruits with soft skins, absorb chemicals and fertilizers easily and therefore might contain high levels of pollution if they are not organic. We suggest that you search for organic, non-genetically modified fruits and grain sweeteners.

Lifestyle Inspirations for Reducing Sugar Cravings

Cravings can act as important information about the things the human body needs. Regular meals that include health-supportive foods that you eat on a daily basis play an important role in balancing cravings. When your sugar cravings are out of the norm, try some of the following.

- Drink a glass of water at the first sign of sugar cravings.
- Reduce your salt (yang) use and products containing salt. Reduce or eliminate animal food (yang), as eating these foods can make you crave sweets (yin).
- Reduce your frequent consumption of alcoholic beverages and caffeinated drinks, as these cause dehydration, blood sugar swings, and sleep deprivation.
- Do regular physical activity you enjoy, which helps to balance blood sugar levels and reduce tension. Start easy and build up to a workout program that you like and can keep up.
- Monitor psychological and emotional triggers. Find meaningful social and spiritual activities and an inspiring career.
- Give and receive massages to bring sweet nourishment into your life.
- Sleep longer and deeper, as sleep deprivation can make you crave sugar and caffeine to get energy.
- Omit chemical or artificial sweeteners or flavors, as these can make you crave more sweets.
- Eat more sweet vegetables and fruits in season. Use whole grain malts or maple syrup in your kitchen.
- Add coriander, cinnamon, nutmeg, cloves, and cardamom to your homemade desserts to satisfy your sweet taste buds.
- Avoid eating constantly. Allow yourself to experience hunger and let the stomach rest—you will have better digestion and a healthy appetite.
- Regularly eat three meals per day. If you need a snack between meals, avoid sugary treats and beverages with caffeine, and eat small amounts of seeds or nuts instead.
- Avoid eating three hours before going to sleep.

Recipes for The Sweet Life

Sweet Chocolaty Adzuki Bean Kanten

4 servings

This kanten is made with agar-agar sea vegetable, which is an excellent source of iodine (160 mg per 100 grams). Agar-agar can be used as a vegetarian gelatin substitute in fruit preserves, kanten, aspics, and soups. It can lower cholesterol, is soothing for the intestines, improves digestion, and is helpful to relieve constipation. See Step 6 for further information.

Ingredients:
4 cups apple juice or half water/half juice
1 cup cooked adzuki beans, mashed
½ cup raisins, or dried fruits of your choice, soaked in juice for 30 minutes
Pinch sea salt
Handful dark chocolate, grated (optional)
4 tbsp. agar-agar flakes (or 2 tbsp. flakes and 2 tbsp. arrowroot/cold water mix)
Topping: your choice of fruit compote
Garnish: mint leaves or another of your choice

Preparation:
1. In a pot, bring apple juice, adzuki bean mash, soaked and drained raisins, and a pinch of sea salt to a boil. (For the bean recipe, see Step 3.)
2. Reduce heat. If using chocolate, stir in and let dissolve.
3. Gradually stir in the agar-agar flakes or the agar-arrowroot mix. The firmness of the kanten depends on the amount of agar-agar used. (The agar-arrowroot mix often provides a smoother texture.)
4. Simmer for about 5 minutes, or until agar-agar completely dissolves, stirring occasionally. It is ready when droplets form on a spoon lifted out of the mixture.
5. Pour into individual molds and add fruit compote of your choice. Or pour into a larger flat serving dish and add fruit compote of your choice.
6. Let cool on the counter or refrigerate until firm, about 45–60 minutes.
7. To serve, top individual servings with a mint leaf or other garnish.

Variations:
- Instead of adzuki beans, use black beans.
- Add a variety of ground seeds or nuts to the dish.
- For an even sweeter taste, add barley or rice malt (contains gluten), rice syrup, or maple syrup before adding agar-agar.
- *Another kanten dish idea:* In a serving dish, alternate cooked mashed squash, cooked mashed chestnuts, and cooked mashed adzuki beans. Top with a cooked apple juice agar-agar mix. Cool for 60 minutes before serving.

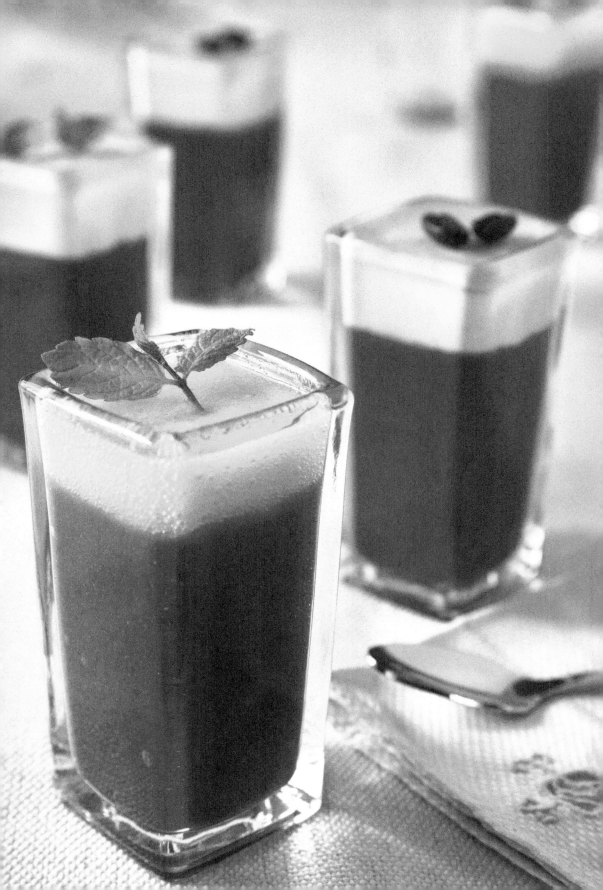

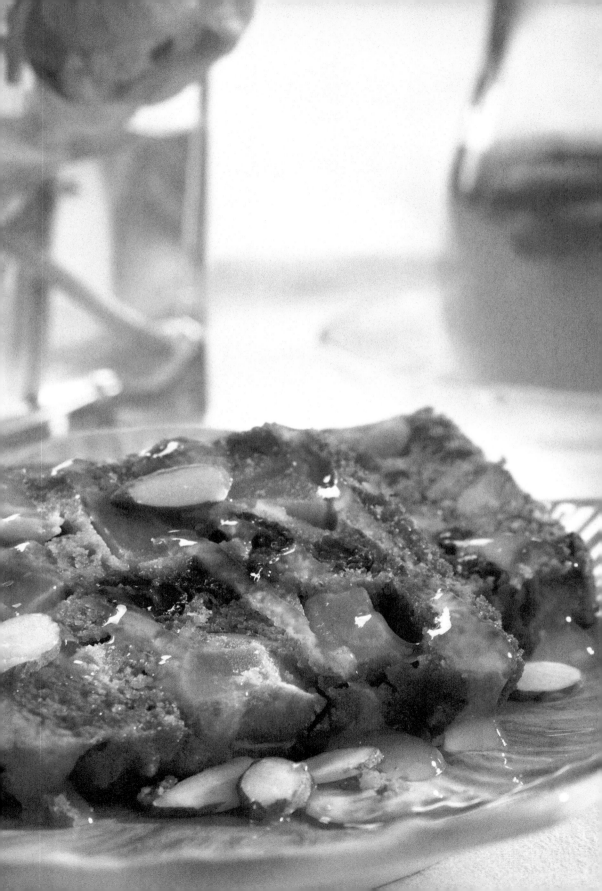

Fruit-Nut Cake with Maple Sauce and Almonds

1 cake

This delicious confection is lovely at teatime. It is reminiscent of many traditional, seasonal European recipes, especially when dried fruits are soaked in rum for one month before adding to the mix.

<u>Wet ingredients</u>:

½ cup high-oleic safflower oil
½ cup maple syrup
½ cup apple juice, or as needed
3 tbsp. applesauce, or as needed
4 oz. soft tofu, pureed
1 tsp. natural vanilla extract, or to taste
2 apples, peeled and cut into cubes
½ cup raisins, soaked in juice (or rum), then drained

<u>Dry ingredients</u>:

2 cups teff and rice flour mix
½ cup rolled oats (gluten free)
2 handfuls slivered almonds, toasted
Pinch sea salt
2–3 tbsp. non-aluminum baking powder
1 tsp. Ceylon cinnamon

<u>Preparation</u>:

1. Preheat oven to 350° F. Lightly oil and flour a loaf pan.
2. Mix wet ingredients together in a bowl. Mix dry ingredients in a large bowl.
3. Slowly fold wet ingredients into dry ingredients until batter is smooth; do not over mix.
4. Adjust the ingredients if necessary, as the batter should be thick and spoonable, not runny.
5. Bake the cake at 350° F for 40–45 minutes. Test with a toothpick for doneness.
6. Cool cake in pan for 10 minutes before removing from pan onto a wire rack.
7. Slice into equal pieces.
8. Serve with *Maple Sauce and Almonds* (or your choice of topping)

Maple Sauce and Almonds: Bring 2 cups of apple juice and a pinch of sea salt to a boil. Reduce to simmer and add 2 tsp. maple syrup. Mix 3 tsp. of kuzu or arrowroot dissolved in 4 tsp. cold water, add to the liquid, and stir constantly until the mixture thickens. Spoon mixture over desserts and garnish with toasted almond slices.

Cranberry Tangerine Sauce

4 servings

Eat this sauce especially during the fall and winter season as a tart-tasting dessert. Use it as a traditional side dish with the *Stuffed Pumpkin–A Possible Holiday Affair* recipe in Step 4. Cranberries have a yang energy compared to strawberries or raspberries (yin), which are tasty during the hotter seasons. Cranberries can also be eaten for bladder discomfort.

Ingredients:
1 cup cranberries
1 cup tangerines, sliced
Tangerine zest, minced
¼ cup apple juice
1/3 cup pure maple syrup
Pinch sea salt
2 tsp. arrowroot or kuzu, dissolved in 5 tsp. of cold water

Preparation:
1. Bring cranberries, fruit juice, maple syrup, and sea salt to a boil in a pan.
2. Stir in the tangerines with the zest.
3. Add the dissolved arrowroot or kuzu and stir till it thickens. (Add just enough to thicken the sauce for your taste.)
4. Serve hot, cold, or room temperature, alone as a dessert, or as a tart side dish.

Variations:
- Add ginger juice to the mix.
- Mix in a variety of other fresh seasonal or dried fruits.
- Instead of maple syrup, use gluten free rice syrup.
- Make it a pie filling: add more arrowroot or kuzu, pour into a piecrust, and bake.

Sweet Grain Amazake Pudding with Strawberries

3 servings

Amazake, a fermented sweet grain drink and natural sweetener that is available in natural food stores, is used to create this pudding. Find ways to include amazake in desserts instead of other sweeteners. Serve it diluted with water as a drink, cold or hot, and occasionally add a pinch of fresh grated ginger juice. Nursing mothers can enjoy drinking it to increase breast milk.

Ingredients:
1 cup amazake (rice or millet)
1 tbsp. arrowroot or kuzu, diluted with 2 tbsp. of cold water
1 cup strawberries, cleaned and quartered
Garnish: lightly toasted crushed nuts

Preparation:

1. Heat the amazake in a small pot and add the diluted arrowroot or kuzu, stirring constantly till it thickens to a cream.
2. Add the strawberries—save some for garnish—and stir gently for half a minute.
3. Serve warm or cool in bowls and garnish with fresh strawberries and toasted nuts.

Variations:

- Instead of amazake, use mashed leftover rice cooked in apple juice.
- Omit strawberries and add a dash of fresh lemon juice and zest, or orange juice and zest, or any fruit of your choice.

Cashew Maple Whip Cream

4 servings

A dash of your own homemade vegan whip cream instead of dairy whipped cream on your desserts can be a surprising delight for guests and family. Serve it with fresh fruit for a quick dessert, or top off cakes, pies, or any favorite sweet course.

Ingredients:

1 cup raw cashews
Filtered or spring water
Vanilla extract, to taste
1 tbsp. maple syrup, or to taste
Garnish: sliced cashews, toasted or raw

Preparation:

1. Wash cashews, and then soak in cold-water overnight.
2. Drain and rinse, but reserve soaking water.
3. In blender or food processor, blend nuts and some of their soaking water until the desired creamy consistency is reached. Add more water if needed.
4. Add vanilla and maple syrup to taste; continue blending and sampling until desired taste is achieved.
5. Garnish with lightly toasted or raw cashew slivers.
6. Leftovers can be refrigerated in a glass container for about 4 days or frozen in serving-size amounts.

Variation:

- Blend in berries or other fruits.

Sweet Cherry-Apple Gluten-Free Crunch

4–6 servings

Prepare this quick and easy dessert any time, as it is easier to make than a fruit pie. Apples and cherries make this crunch a colorful and flavorsome dish. It will become a favorite, and you can make any variations you like.

Filling ingredients:

1. 2–3 cups baking apples, cored and diced
2. Lemon juice to coat the apples
3. 1 cup sweet cherries, fresh or frozen, seeds removed, sliced
4. Small pinch sea salt

Topping dry ingredients:

1. 1 cup teff flour or brown rice flour
2. 1–2 cups quinoa flakes or rice flakes, or gluten-free oat flakes
3. ½ cup hazelnuts (or other nuts), lightly toasted and slivered
4. ½ tsp. Ceylon cinnamon
5. ¼ cup dark chocolate, slivered (optional)

Topping wet ingredients:

1. ¼ –½ cup coconut oil or high-oleic safflower oil
    1 cup maple syrup
2. Filtered or spring water, small amount, if needed

Preparation:

1. Preheat oven to 350° F.
2. Place diced apples in a baking dish and mix with lemon juice to stop oxidization.
3. Toss with a pinch of sea salt and add the cherries.
4. Optional: quickly toast flour and flakes for a nuttier flavor.
5. In a bowl, mix dry ingredients. Add half of the chocolate now, if using, and the rest toward end of baking time.
6. In a separate container, mix oil and syrup with a fork.
7. Add the wet to the dry ingredients and combine with fork or hand to form small clumps. Add a few drops of water, if needed.
8. Spread topping evenly over the fruit mix.
9. Add a small amount of water to the baking dish and cover with parchment paper and then (optional) foil.
10. Bake covered 30–45 minutes and then uncovered 15–20 minutes.
11. Toward the end of baking, sprinkle rest of dark chocolate over the topping, if using, and let it melt into the topping.
12. Serve as is or with *Cashew Maple Whip Cream* from this Step.

Variations:

*   Use other seasonal fruits, like strawberries, raspberries, blueberries, pears, or peaches.
*   If you are not baking for people with gluten sensitivities, you could substitute whole-wheat pastry flour for the teff or rice flour.

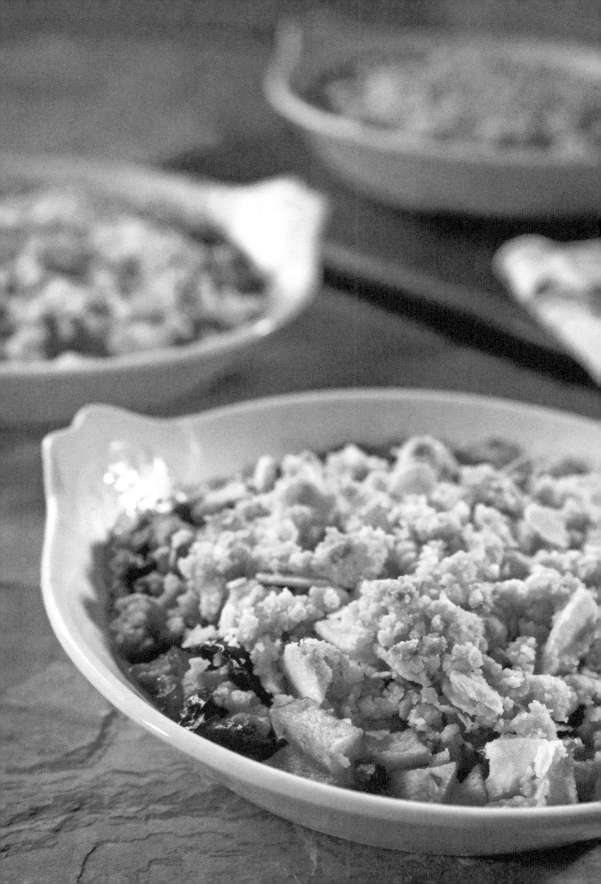

Warm Vanilla Sauce

Adjustable servings

Use this sauce warm over your favorite desserts.

Ingredients:
2 cups non-dairy milk
6 tsps. almond butter
6 tbsp. rice syrup or maple syrup
Natural vanilla extract, to taste
Pinch lemon zest, or to taste
3 tbsp. arrowroot or kuzu, dissolved in 5 tbsp. cold water

Preparation:
1. Bring non-dairy milk, almond butter, and syrup to a boil. Stir till almond butter is dissolved.
2. Turn heat down, stir in arrowroot or kuzu liquid, simmer and stir until sauce has thickened.
3. Stir in lemon zest and vanilla.
4. Eat warm over fruits or cakes.

Gluten-Free Raspberry Cookie

2 dozen

This is a very yummy and healthy cookie.

Dry ingredients:
2 cups walnut flour, or grind nuts in a food processor
1½ cups quinoa flakes (or flour)
3 cups brown rice flour
1 tbsp. cinnamon
Pinch sea salt

Wet ingredients:
¾ cup rice syrup
¾ cup maple syrup
½ cup organic high-oleic safflower oil, chilled
½ cup organic soy or rice milk
2 tsp. vanilla extract
10-ounce jar fruit-sweetened raspberry jam

Preparation:
1. Preheat oven to 355º F.
2. With a food processor or fork, combine dry ingredients to make a medium-fine meal.
3. Whisk together the wet ingredients in a large mixing bowl.

4. Add the dry ingredients to the wet ingredients and mix thoroughly.
5. Allow the dough to rest for 10–15 minutes to firm up.
6. Line cookie sheets with parchment paper.
7. Form the cookie dough into 2-inch balls and place them on the cookie sheets.
8. In the center of each ball, make a well with your thumb or a small spoon and add about a teaspoon and a half of raspberry jam.
9. Bake about 20 minutes, or until crisp on top and light golden brown on the bottom.
10. Cool on the pans for 5 minutes or so before removing to wire racks to finish cooling.

Variations:

If you are not baking for people with gluten sensitivities, you could substitute rolled oats (ground in a food processor) for the quinoa flakes, and whole-wheat pastry flour for the rice flour.

Breakfast or anytime recipes

Mochi-Sweet Rice Puff

4–6 pieces per person

Mochi is made from sweet rice that has been simmered and pounded into a flat cake. It can be bought in blocks ready-made. Mochi has a nice sweet taste and is helpful in overcoming anemia and general fatigue, and for gaining weight. Nursing mothers can enjoy it to increase breast milk. It has an amazing ability to puff up and take on a delightfully chewy texture when heated.

Ingredients:

1 tsp. high-oleic safflower oil
1 block sweet rice mochi
Garnish: drizzles of gluten free rice or maple syrup (optional)
Garnish: slices of nori sea vegetables and tamari/water mix

Preparation:

1. Heat oil in a skillet. Stainless steel is OK, but cast iron is best.
2. Cut mochi into 2-inch cubes and place into the skillet. Cover and reduce heat.
3. Cook each side until lightly browned. Check often.
4. Cover, and continue cooking on low until the pieces puff up and expand. This could take 5 to 10 minutes.
5. Serve warm, with optional drizzle of rice or maple syrup, or wrap a slice of nori around each piece and dip into a tamari/water mixture.

Variations:

*   Bake on a lightly oiled pan in a 350° F preheated oven until it puffs and browns.
*   Garnish the cooked mochi with fresh or cooked fruit.
*   Top with *Cashew Maple Whip Cream* from this book.
*   Add a few pieces of plain cooked mochi to your miso soup.

Gluten-Free Crepes

Adjustable servings

Crepes are thinner versions of pancakes. They are a popular and welcome addition to your kitchen from the French cuisine.

Ingredients:

1 cup gluten-free baking flour mix or a mix of garbanzo bean flour, potato starch, tapioca flour, white sorghum flour, fava bean flour
1/8 tsp. sea salt (a bit more for savory crepes)
1 cup sparkling water, cold (more or less according to desired thickness)
High-oleic safflower or grapeseed oil, as needed

Optional fillings:

Savory: mushrooms and sautéed onions, or greens with finely grated mochi
Sweet: grated chocolate and/or fresh strawberries, or jelly.

Preparation:

1. Mix salt, flour, and sparkling water. Whisk until smooth. Make sure all lumps are gone.
2. Brush a flat cast iron skillet with oil and heat.
3. Pour a medium-sized circle of batter onto the skillet. Immediately spread into a thin disc using a crepe spreader, or lift the pan and tilt to spread it into a larger circle.
4. Heat until the edges just begin to lightly lift or become crisp (about a minute or less).
5. Turn the crepe and cook on the other side for another minute or so, depending on the thickness of the crepe. The crepes should be soft.
6. Remove from heat, and place on a plate with a towel over them to keep them warm.
7. Brush skillet with oil again, and repeat the process until all batter is used.
8. Before serving, place each crepe back on the warm skillet. Spread with a sweet or savory filling in a half circle. Fold crepe in half, then quarters. Remove from heat and serve immediately.
9. Tip: If you make them ahead, be sure to store in an airtight container or they will dry out.

*   **Optional garnish:** a spoonful of *Cashew Maple Whip Cream.*

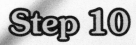

Step 10

Kitchen Remedies, Tonics, and Therapies

"Let food be thy medicine and medicine be thy food."

Hippocrates

For centuries, homespun tonics, remedies, and healing therapies have been passed down from one generation to the next. So it's likely that some are already in your hands. With this Step, we share our favorite macrobiotic therapies, remedies, and tinctures for you to include in your repertoire. These remedies and healing methods are based on traditional medicines and spiritual teachings of China and Japan, as well as Europe and the rest of the world. Historically, they have been used to alleviate various lifestyle and food imbalances. For deeper studies and background, refer to the book *Macrobiotic Home Remedies: Your Guide To Traditional Healing Techniques.*

Food is medicine, and using specific home remedies is a great way to maximize the healing potential of various food items. Just a few ingredients in careful combinations can support beneficial changes in your health. For instance, think ginger or cayenne pepper when you have lung congestion, and stay away from dairy products, as these produce mucus and aggravate the condition.

Recent research shows how important it is to eat balanced meals that include all food groups in order to obtain the nutrients the body needs. The external and internal home therapies in this Step are helpful in creating balance during distress or during the seasonal changes. Note that these kitchen remedies, drinks, tonics, and therapies don't take the place of the advice of a medical doctor and/or a qualified nutritionist.

Kukicha Twig Tea with Umeboshi

This drink helps to strengthen the blood, regulate digestion and circulation, relieve fatigue and weakness, and provide relief from an overconsumption of simple sugars, including fruit, fruit juices, or other acid-forming foods or beverages. Umeboshi is a Japanese-style plum, more like an apricot, which has been pickled in salt, usually with beefsteak leaves (*shiso*).

Ingredients:
½ to 1 umeboshi plum
1 cup hot kukicha tea (boil water and kukicha until the water is light brown, then strain).
Optional: ½–1 tsp. tamari

Preparation:
1. Mash desired amount of plum into a 6 oz. teacup.
2. Add tamari, if using.
3. Pour the hot kukicha tea into the cup and stir well. Drink hot.

Leafy Green Vegetable Tea

This drink is very relaxing and is said to help to loosen stagnated protein and animal fats. Look under Step 1 for the raw *Blended Green Vegetable Drink*.

Ingredients:

Green leafy vegetables, singly or in combination: kale, collards, dandelion, daikon or turnip leaves, or Chinese (Napa) cabbage
Filtered or spring water; Pinch sea salt or a few drops tamari

Preparation:

1. Wash and very finely chop the vegetables.
2. Add twice the amount of water as vegetables.
3. Bring to a gentle boil and simmer for 3–5 minutes.
4. Add a pinch of sea salt or a few drops of tamari toward the end, and stir.
5. Optional: Eat the vegetables with the broth. Or save them for later use in soups or stews.
6. Drink hot or at room temperature.

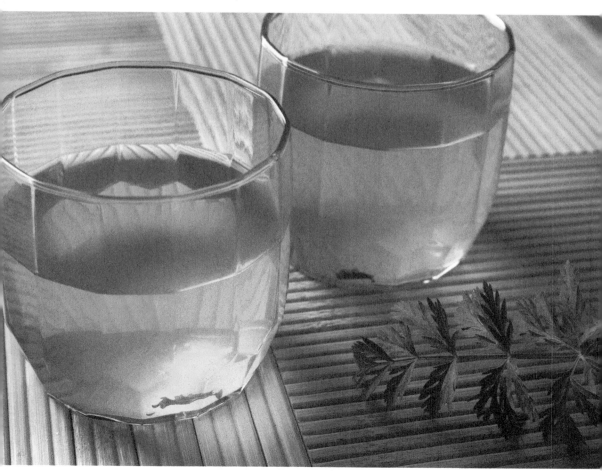

Carrot and Daikon Drink

(Photo p. 189)

This is a classic macrobiotic drink that helps digestion. With repeated use, it can also dissolve solidified fat deposits that exist deep within the body.

Ingredients:
½ cup carrots
½ cup daikon
1 cup filtered or spring water
Few drops tamari
1/3 sheet nori sea vegetable, shredded
½ umeboshi plum

Preparation:
1. Finely grate the carrots and daikon. Bring to a gentle boil with water in a saucepan and simmer for about 3 minutes. Add the nori and umeboshi and continue cooking a few minutes longer. Add a few drops of tamari toward the end.
2. Eat the vegetables and drink the broth.

Relaxing Sweet Vegetable Drink

1-2 cups per day

For a strong body and mind, we often suggest juicing with vegetables and minimizing fruit juicing. Fruit juices are high in antioxidants, including vitamin C, and can provide relief during times of distress. However, fruit sugars (as well as other sugars) have been shown to depress the immune system. Drink this instead of a sweet fruit juice, as it does not create blood sugar spikes.

Ingredients:
½ cup onions (optional)
½ cup carrots
½ cup green cabbage
½ cup sweet winter squash
6-8 cups filtered or spring water

Preparation:
- Clean vegetables and finely chop, or use a blender or food processor.
- Place vegetables into a pot, add the water, and bring to a boil for 2–3 minutes.
- Reduce flame to low, cover, and simmer for 20 minutes.
- Strain the broth.
- Optional: Eat the vegetables with the broth. Or save them for later use in soups or stews.
- Drink the broth either warm or at room temperature.
- Keep in the refrigerator, but warm again or return to room temperature before drinking.

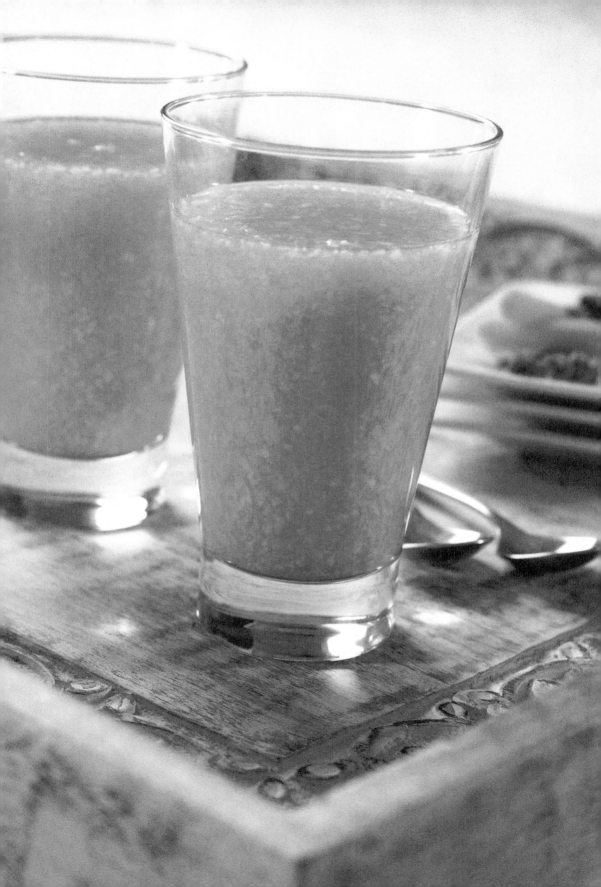

Variations:

- Use a variety of sweet-tasting root and round vegetables like red beets, red cabbage, daikon, turnips, celery root, and rutabaga.
- Add greens towards the end of cooking.

Liver Revitalizing Tea

Use this tea especially during the spring season to revitalize your liver, or any time you feel tense and tight, or have eaten too many fatty foods. Michio Kushi developed this liver tonic tea during the first Level 4 seminars he conducted at the Kushi Institute in Becket, Massachusetts.

Ingredients:
2 parts unroasted buckwheat groats
2 parts sprouts (mung bean, alfalfa, soy, or any other)
1 part shiitake mushroom, dried and soaked

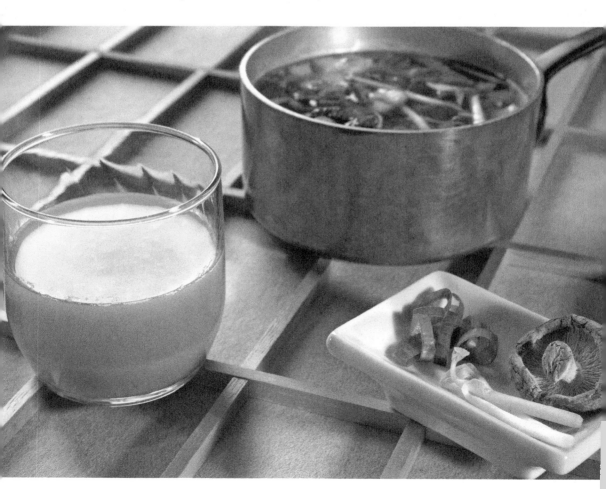

1 part daikon
2 parts daikon greens (or turnip, radish, or collard greens)
1 part scallion
5 times more filtered water than total volume of other ingredients

Preparation:
1. Chop all vegetables and combine all ingredients in a large pot.
2. Add water. Bring to a boil, lower the flame, and simmer for about 30 minutes.
3. Strain and drink the tea during the day.

Digestive Tonics and Drinks

Feelings of fatigue or bloating after a meal can be signs that your system has difficulty assimilating your food. Many of the home remedies in this Step can enhance your digestion. But there are other methods that support a strong digestive system.
- Prepare your food properly, including soaking your grains and beans before cooking.
- Don't drink cold beverages while you eat.
- Eat smaller portion sizes and chew more. Count to 30 or even 50. The enzyme alpha-amylase in your saliva starts to break down carbohydrates, and the enzyme lingual lipase contributes to the earliest stages of the digestion of fat.
- Drink one or two cups of miso soup daily.
- With each meal, add one tablespoon of pickles or other lactic acid-fermented products. Review Step 5 for recipes.
- In certain cases, supplementation with food-based enzymes, probiotics, and prebiotics might also be helpful.

Vitamin and Mineral Therapy

Established requirements and recommendations for vitamins and minerals vary depending on age, gender, and activity, and for women, lactation, pregnancy, or menopausal status. Sources of vitamins and minerals are also varied. One cup of cooked collard greens contains 300 mg of calcium, the same amount as one cup of dairy milk. Stay away from artificially processed calcium-fortified soymilk, or calcium-processed tofu.

Always have a balanced seasonal meal plan ready to support your vitamin and mineral needs. If you take supplements for one reason or another, choose food-based vegan vitamins and sea or lake vegetable-based mineral supplements like chlorella. Eat a toasted sheet of nori sea vegetable daily, or use macrobiotic condiments like gomasio (recipe in Step 8) to support your efforts to lead a healthy, long life.

Use small amounts of fresh seasonal fruit and raw or pickled vegetables (see Step 6) to supplement your vitamins that are not heat resistant like vitamin C, which may be destroyed in cooking. It is also important to spend 15–20 minutes outdoors in the sun daily to get vitamin D. Eat foods like sundried daikon, lotus root, burdock, and sea vegetables that are rich in Vitamin D.

Herbal Tea Therapy

Most cultures around the world, such as Vedic, Amazonian, Native American, Tibetan, European, and Chinese, have their own herbal folklore and plant medicines. Herbal medicines can be wonderful therapeutic additions to your natural kitchen. A wide variety of healing herbs can be used in tinctures or teas by steeping dried or fresh herbs in hot water. See Step 7, *Beverages and Soups for All Seasons* for further digestive, immune enhancing, and stimulating herbal teas.

Nettle Tea

Nettle tea can support your immune system, especially during allergy season. Early spring is a great time to pick fresh, nourishing nettles, as these are one of the first plants that peek out of the ground after the snow has disappeared. Their tender top shoots can be picked for food until the nettle begins to flower, about one or two months later. Collect plenty and dry them to make a tea or tincture by steeping them in hot water.[110]

Mu Tea

Mu tea is based on traditional Chinese herbal medicine and was developed by George Ohsawa, founder of macrobiotics. It is available in sixteen-herb and nine-herb formulations of plants and wild herbs. Both teas are good for digestive and respiratory functions and are traditionally known to be particularly helpful for female problems. Although both teas include yin and yang ingredients, the sixteen-herb version results in an overall more yang drink. Mu tea is available in natural food stores or online.

Macrobiotic Water Therapy

You can use water therapy internally and externally. For an internal water cleanse, drink one cup of warm filtered or spring water in the morning before drinking anything or eating breakfast. Externally, use a water compress or a steam bath in various wellness therapies. A ginger compress can loosen stagnant energy in your body and assist you in stimulating circulation. A daily *hot water body scrub*, with or without ginger, will support the cleansing of your biggest organ—your skin.

Hot Water Body Scrub

This scrub helps to activate circulation, and it aids the lymphatic system, especially when scrubbing the underarm and groin areas. The daily hot water scrub also promotes clear and clean skin, as it helps discharge fat that has accumulated under the skin, and opens skin pores in order to promote smooth and regular elimination of any excess fat and toxins. Another benefit is the relief of stress and muscle tension through the meditative action of rubbing the skin. For best results, do the hot water body scrub once or twice daily, in the morning and/or at night, before or after a shower or bath—or any time during the day.

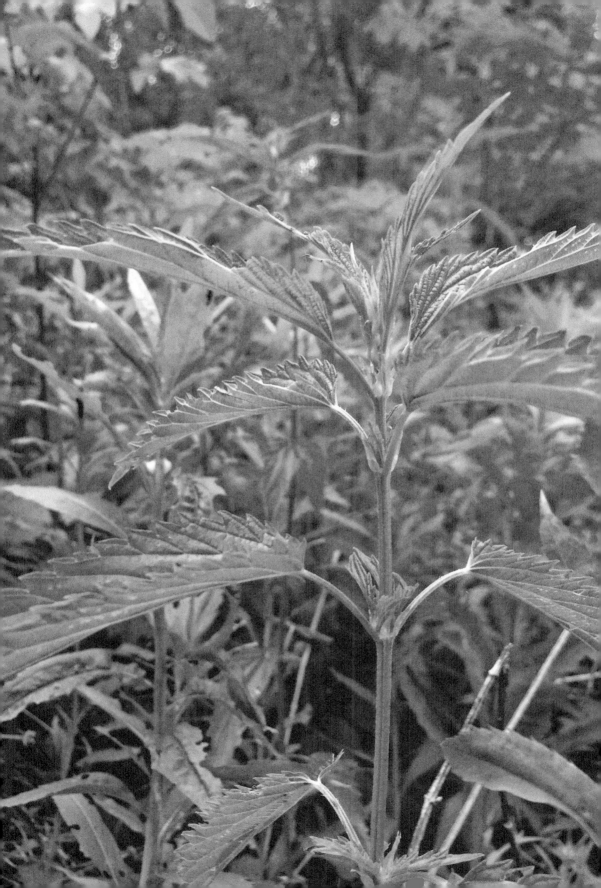

Ingredients:

Hot filtered water

Preparation:

1. Fill sink with hot water.
2. Dip central portion of a small cotton towel or cloth in the water, holding it at both ends.
3. Wring out excess water.
4. Scrub the whole body, repeatedly dipping towel or cloth into the hot water when it cools down. Do one section of the body at a time: for example, begin with the hands and fingers and work your way up the arms to the shoulders, neck, and face. Start with your toes, feet, legs, and buttocks; lower back, upper back and then the chest.
5. The skin should become pink or slightly red. This result may take a few days to achieve if the skin is clogged with accumulated fats.

Variation:

• Squeeze the juice from a handful of finely grated ginger into the hot water.

Sea Vegetable Therapy Bath

A sea vegetable bath warms the body. In addition, it aids in extracting body odors caused by the consumption of animal foods. It can also draw out excess fat and oil from the body and clear up skin problems. It is best and most effective just before bedtime, but at least one hour after eating. This bath, also called *Hip Bath,* is specifically good for women's reproductive organs (see Variation). It is similar to thalassotherapy, a process developed in the nineteenth century in Brittany that uses seawater and sea products combined with mud.

Ingredients:

Handful of dried arame sea vegetable
4–5 quarts filtered or spring water
Sea salt

Preparation:

1. Place a handful of arame sea vegetables in a large pot.
2. Add about four to five quarts of water and bring to a boil.
3. Reduce to a medium flame and simmer until the water is brown.
4. Add approximately one cup of sea salt to the pot and stir well to dissolve.
5. Strain and pour the hot liquid into a small tub.
6. Add hot water until bath level is hip or waist high when sitting in the tub.
7. Keep the temperature as hot as possible and cover your upper body with a large towel to induce perspiration.
8. Stay in the bath for 10–20 minutes, until the hip area becomes very red and hot.
9. Keep the hip area warm after coming out of the bath.

Variation:

When the *Hip Bath* is used for women's reproductive organs, arame is helpful, but you could also use 4 or 5 bunches of dried daikon leaves or turnip leaves instead of arame. Dry your own fresh daikon leaves or turnip leaves in a shady place and store for this use.

Therapeutic Macrobiotic Plasters and Bandages

Tofu Plaster

The tofu plaster is traditionally known to help with concussions, hemorrhoids, fevers, and burns. In many cases it is more effective than ice, as it retains a cool temperature for longer periods.

Ingredients:
1 block organic tofu
Unbleached white flour (10–20% of tofu volume)
Grated ginger (5% of tofu volume)

Preparation:
1. Mash tofu in a suribachi or with a fork or hand. Squeeze out and discard the liquid.
2. Add flour and grated ginger. Mix well.
3. Apply the mixture directly to the skin or wrap it in cheesecloth.
4. Cover with a towel. You may want to secure it in place with a bandage or tie with a cotton strip.
5. Change the plaster every 2–3 hours or when it becomes hot. Use until condition betters.

Kombu Bandage

The kombu bandage is good for burns from radiation, skin lesions, and scars.

Preparation:
Soak strips of kombu (the length depends on the area to be covered) and cut to proper size, enough for a double layer.
Apply the soaked kombu to the affected area, directly on the skin, in double layers. Cover with a cotton cloth and leave on for three hours or longer. You may want to secure it in place with a bandage or tie with a cotton strip.

Visualization

In your mind's eye, travel inside your body to the place where you don't feel well. When you reach it, perform a healing ritual by imagining light coming to that place. Do this visualization two times a day for fifteen minutes during distress.

Self-Massage

Massaging one's own hands and feet is something everybody can do. Fingers and toes are connected through energy lines to all the organs of the body, and massaging your digits helps to energize your whole body.

The Do-In exercise and body self-massage system[111] is a great way to activate your whole body's meridian system and muscles. Make a fist with each hand and tap lightly on one section of the body at a time. For example, begin with the hands and fingers and work your way up the arms to the shoulders, neck, and face. Then go up from your toes, feet, legs, buttocks, lower back, abdomen, upper back, and then the chest. The skin should become slightly pink, and you might feel warm.

Aromatherapy

The aromas of plants have been used in the healing arts for centuries. Some ancient Ayurveda texts, like the *Rig Veda,* describe sophisticated methods used as long as 5,000 years ago for concentrating aromas. Essential oils for aromatherapy nowadays are extracted from plant materials by applying steam to force out their essences into highly concentrated liquids.

Choose essential oils that fit your needs and that assist you in feeling good. Start with lavender (yin), as it is one of the most versatile oils. Besides its beautiful aroma, it has antibacterial properties and is calming and sedative, helping promote deep relaxation and sleep. For essential oils that invigorate (yang), choose ginger, rosemary, or sage.

How to apply essential oils:

* Use a few drops on your wrist or in your hand. Rub your palms together and inhale the aroma right from your hands.
* Add just a few drops to a bowl of hot water and use a towel to rub it over your body.
* Add a few drops to your bath water.

Peaceful Breathing

Breathing exercises are easy, as everybody is breathing already. For meditative and relaxing purposes, try the following breathing exercise: Breathe in for 4 counts, then hold your breath for 4 counts and breathe out for 6 counts. Do this simple breathing exercise for 5 minutes, 3–4 times a day, for a peaceful, meditative mind.[112]

Bringing It All Together

We'd like to thank you, our reader, for taking the time to read this book that we have put so much of our hearts into. We hope that you are inspired to take your knowledge into the kitchen and practice with it.

We are aware that learning to choose and prepare new foods in new ways can be a bit daunting at first, which is why we chose to break it all down into Steps for you. Rest assured that it will soon become easier and even feel like second nature to you. Your kitchen work will be more intuitive, and what at first seemed laborious will become fun and exciting as you discover new tastes and textures that change with the seasons. As your skills develop, you will start surprising yourself with all of your accomplishments and discoveries.

If you already eating in season or have studied macrobiotics before, this book will refresh you with up-to-date information and provide support to continue on your path.

The macrobiotic way of life is a conscious way of living in harmony with nature, your environment, climate zone, and seasons. It is like a dance in which you learn to balance these ever-changing natural forces. For instance, even though blueberries and brown rice are wonderful foods and you might think it is good to eat them every day all year long, that would not be eating in season. On the other hand, it would be better to eat these foods out of season rather than daily sugary treats. We would call that way of eating a transitional macrobiotic way.

Even so, a macrobiotic kitchen allows for a very flexible lifestyle with a wide variety of food choices. In this book we have followed the standard macrobiotic diet pyramid for temperate regions, with proportional food guidelines. This way you can start eating and cooking right away, without having to take the time to study yin and yang in depth. These standard guidelines will apply to a transitional macrobiotic kitchen, seasonal kitchen, age and gender appropriate kitchen, and so forth. They will also apply to a healing or convalescent lifestyle, but for these you should, in addition, contact a certified macrobiotic counselor.

To make your macrobiotic life easier, we have included a general balanced weekly menu plan. You can adapt the recipes with ingredients appropriate to your region, according to the seasons. As different cultures eat their main meal at different times, we have put lunch and dinner menus together. We advise you to cook enough for several meals to save time and have enough left over to pack a meal to go for you and your family when you are away from home.

We have shown you a way to a peaceful and healthy life. It's now your choice to start taking the Steps, one or more at a time, to suit your own pace. Keep this book in your kitchen and refer often to the recipes and charts. We suggest a food journal so you can easily monitor your experiments—and your successes--as you make your way through all Ten Steps.

We extend our warmest wishes to you and your loved ones, and we hope that this book will be the best kitchen tool you have ever picked up.

Gabriele Kushi and Michio Kushi

Appendix

Staples for Your Macrobiotic Kitchen

Stock your pantry shelves with all the provisions you learned about in this book. You want to have them handy whenever you need them. This is a great step to a healthy natural foods and macrobiotic kitchen. Store grains, beans, sea vegetables, mushrooms, seeds, nuts, and dried fruits in glass containers and label them for easy access. Opt always for non-genetically modified food, and get organically grown foods and traditionally made products whenever possible. Natural food stores, ethnic markets, cooperatives, farmers' markets, some grocery stores, and on-line stores offer the best quality food.

Beans: Adzuki beans, black soybeans, chickpeas (garbanzos), lentils (green, brown, yellow, red)

Bean Products: Tempeh, tofu (fresh and dried), natto

Beverages: Bancha tea (roasted leaves), barley grain coffee (contains gluten), green tea with brown rice (or other versions), kukicha tea (roasted stems), red tea

Condiments: Gomasio (sesame sea salt mix), nori flakes, shiso leaves and powder, tekka

Cookware: Wooden cutting board and utensils, graters (ceramic and metal), pickle press, pots and pans (stainless steel, glass, ceramic, cast iron), pressure cooker, suribachi and pestle, sushi mat (bamboo), vegetable knife (MAC© or other good Japanese brand)

Grains—Whole, Gluten-Free: Amaranth, brown rice (short, medium, long grain), corn, Hato mugi (wild barley, Job's tears), millet, oats (prepared in a gluten-free facility), quinoa, sweet rice, wild rice

Grains—Whole, Gluten-Containing: Barley, kamut, spelt, einkorn, emmer (farro)

Nuts: Almonds, chestnuts, walnuts, hazelnuts

Oils: Flax (raw with lignans), nut oils, olive oil (cold-pressed extra virgin), sesame oils (unrefined light and dark-roasted)

Pickles: Ginger pickles, homemade pickles, raw sauerkraut, takuan daikon radish pickle

Seasonings: Kuzu; arrowroot; mirin; miso—aged 3 months: light, mellow rice, chickpea; and miso aged 1-2+ years: rice, adzuki, barley (contains gluten); black pepper; Himalayan salt; sea salt (white or unbleached); soy sauce (contains gluten); tamari (wheat-free soy sauce); umeboshi (plum, paste); vinegars (umeboshi, rice, apple cider)

Sea Vegetables: Agar-agar (kanten), arame, dulse flakes, hijiki, kombu, nori (sushi style and flakes), sea palm, wakame flakes and strands

Seeds: Chia, flax, hemp, pumpkin, sesame, sunflower

Sweeteners: Amazake, apple juice, barley malt (contains gluten), brown rice malt (contains gluten), brown rice syrup, green stevia (green liquid), maple syrup

Menu Suggestions for One Week

	Monday	Tuesday	Wednesday	Thursday	Friday	Saturday	Sunday	Other Options
Breakfast	Kukicha tea Soft grain porridge with nori condiment or fruit	Green tea Toast with jam	Coffee or Tea Scrambled tofu with seasonal vegetables	Kukicha tea Sweet-tasting carrot and squash puree	Green tea Black bean burrito with mango salsa	Blended green vegetable drink Seasonal fruits	Coffee or Tea Crepes	Miso soup Seasonal fruits Soft grains Steamed greens
Snack	Seeds, 1/4 cup	Raw veggies crudités with avocado and basil dip	Seasonal fruits	Kale chips	Nuts, 1/4 cup	Dessert from Step 9	Edamame or Steamed green beans	Specialty drinks Pack snacks ahead for the week
Dinner/Lunch	Boiled whole grain brown rice with gomasio Green leafy vegetable roll Smoky black-peppered seared green beans	Miso soup with greens Quinoa salad with sautéed vegetables Tempeh sandwich with greens and root vegetable	Kale with raisins and almonds Grain dish of your choice Black beans with yellow corn	Miso soup Fried rice patties (made with leftover rice) Steamed greens Three bean salad	Nabe style vegetables Pan-roasted millet with mushroom sauce Sprouted mung bean salad with lemon dressing	Mystic miso greens with daikon radish Buckwheat noodles with ginger/scallions Lentils	Wild rice and vegetable sauté Kale with golden raisins and toasted almond slivers Nori-wrapped tofu with miso	Add small side servings from one or more of the following: Pickles (Step 5) Pressed Salad (Steps 3 and 5) Condiments (Step 8) Sea Vegetables (Step 6)

Macrobiotic Dietary Guidelines
for Temperate Regions

including North America, Europe, Russia, China, East Asia, and Moderate
Regions in Southern Africa,
South America, Australia, and New Zealand

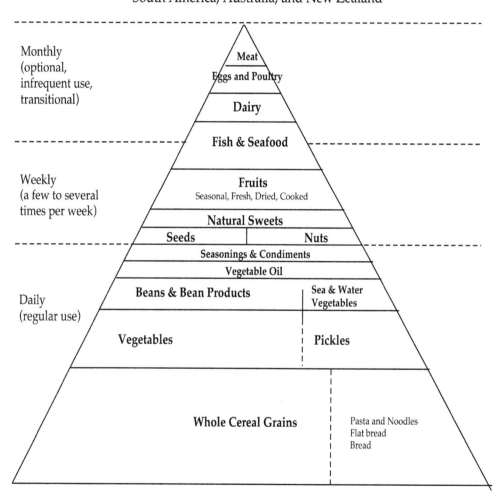

Monthly
(optional,
infrequent use,
transitional)

Weekly
(a few to several
times per week)

Daily
(regular use)

Meat
Eggs and Poultry
Dairy
Fish & Seafood
Fruits
Seasonal, Fresh, Dried, Cooked
Natural Sweets
Seeds   Nuts
Seasonings & Condiments
Vegetable Oil
Beans & Bean Products   Sea & Water Vegetables
Vegetables   Pickles
Whole Cereal Grains   Pasta and Noodles
Flat bread
Bread

Macrobiotic Dietary Guidelines
for Temperate Regions
including North America, Europe, Russia, China, East Asia,
and Moderate Regions in Southern Africa,
South America, Australia, and New Zealand

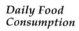

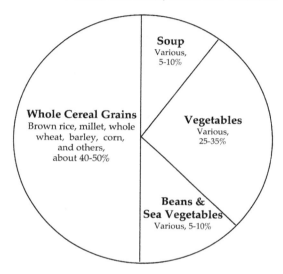

Plus supplemental foods and beverages:
Fish and seafood (optional)
Local fruit, seeds, and nuts
Natural processed oils, seasonings, and condiments,
Natural sweets
Non-aromatic and nonstimulant beverages and
occasional aromatic and stimulant beverages

Food to be organically grown as much as possible
Water to be spring, well, or purified
Fire to be from wood, charcoal, gas, solar, or other
natural source

Glossary of Terms

Adzuki Bean: Small, dark red bean, grown originally in Japan but now also grown in the West. Also known as aduki bean.

Amazake: A sweet, creamy beverage made from fermented sweet brown rice.

Arame: A thin, wiry, black, mineral-rich sea vegetable, similar to hijiki.

Bancha Tea: Twigs, stems, and leaves from mature Japanese tea bushes; also known as *kukicha* tea.

Barley: A whole cereal grain and traditional staple of the Middle East and Southern Europe. It contains gluten.

Barley Malt: A natural sweetener made from concentrated barley that has a rich, roasted taste. It contains gluten.

Brown Rice: Whole unpolished rice comes in three main varieties: short, medium, and long grain. Brown rice contains an ideal balance of nutrients and is the principal staple in macrobiotic cooking.

Cold-Pressed: Pertaining to oils processed at low temperatures to preserve their natural qualities.

Daikon: A long white radish used in many types of dishes and for medicinal purposes.

Dulse: A red-purple sea vegetable used in soups, salads, vegetable dishes, or as a garnish.

Gomasio: Sesame seed salt made from dry roasting and grinding sea salt and sesame seeds and crushing them in a suribachi.

Hijiki: A dark brown sea vegetable which when dried turns black. It has a wiry consistency and may be strong tasting. Grows native to Japan and the North Atlantic.

Kombu: A wide, thick, dark sea vegetable that grows in deep ocean water. Used in making soup stocks, condiments, and candy. It can be cooked as a separate dish or with vegetables, beans, or grains.

Macrobiotics: From the traditional Greek word for Great Life or Long Life, this is the way of life according to the largest possible view—the infinite order of the universe. The practice of macrobiotics includes the understanding and practical application of the order of the universe in daily life. This includes the selection, preparation, and manner of cooking and eating, as well as the orientation of consciousness.

Millet: A small yellow grain that can be prepared whole, added to soups, salads, and vegetable dishes, or baked. It is a staple food of China and Africa.

Mirin: A sweet cooking wine made from sweet rice.

Miso: A fermented paste made from soybeans, sea salt, and usually, rice or barley. Used in soups, stews, spreads, baking, and as seasoning, miso has a nice sweet taste and gives a salty flavor.

Natto: Cooked white soybeans mixed with beneficial enzymes and fermented for twenty-four hours. This is a sticky dish with long strands and a strong odor, and is good for improving digestion.

Natural Foods: Whole foods not processed or treated with artificial additives or preservatives, chemical fertilizers, herbicides, pesticides, genetically modified (GMO) organisms, or other artificial sprays.

Nori: Thin sheets of dried sea vegetables that are black or dark purple and turn green when roasted over a flame. They can be used as a garnish, to wrap rice balls, in making sushi, or with tamari as a condiment.

Organic Foods: Foods grown without the use of chemical fertilizers, herbicides, pesticides, genetically modified (GMO) organisms, or other artificial sprays.

Oxalic Acid: Found in plants; binds with calcium to form insoluble compounds that limit the calcium that can be absorbed.

Pressed Salad: Salad prepared by pressing sliced vegetables and sea salt in a small pickle press or with an improvised weight.

Pressure Cooker: An airtight metal pot that cooks food quickly by steaming it under pressure at high temperature. Used primarily in macrobiotic cooking for whole grains and occasionally for beans with vegetables.

Rice Syrup: A natural sweetener made from malted brown rice. Available gluten-free.

Sea Salt: Salt obtained from the ocean. Unlike refined table salt, unrefined sea salt is high in trace minerals and contains no chemicals, sugar, or added iodine.

Sea Vegetable: Edible mineral-rich vegetable from the seas such as kombu, wakame, arame, hijiki, nori, or dulse.

Shiitake: A mushroom native to Japan but now cultivated in the West as well. Used widely dried or fresh in cooking, for soups and stews, and in medical preparations.

Soba Noodles: Made from 100 % buckwheat flour; is gluten free. Buckwheat noodles made with some whole-wheat flour contain gluten.

Soymilk: The liquid residue from cooking tofu. Used as a beverage, often as a milk substitute.

Soy Foods: Products made from soybeans such as miso, tofu, tempeh, natto, tamari, and soy sauce (contains gluten).

Suribachi: A serrated, glazed clay bowl or mortar. It is used with a wooden pestle called a *surikogi* for grinding and puréeing foods.

Sushi: A traditional Japanese dish consisting of rice seasoned with vinegar and served with various vegetables, sea vegetables, seafood, or pickles. In addition to spiral rounds, sushi can be prepared in several other styles.

Sushi Mat: A small bamboo mat used to roll up nori-maki sushi or vegetables, or to cover bowls and dishes to keep food warm.

Sweet Rice: This rice is slightly sweeter than regular rice and is used in a variety of regular and holiday dishes.

Tahini: A thick, smooth paste made from ground whole sesame seeds.

Tamari: Traditional, naturally made soy sauce, as distinguished from refined, chemically processed soy sauce. Also known as organic or natural shoyo. A stronger, wheat-free soy sauce called real or genuine tamari, a byproduct of making miso, is used for special dishes. Tamari soy sauce is used for daily cooking.

Tekka: Condiment made from hatcho miso, sesame oil, burdock, lotus root, carrot, and ginger root. It is the black powder that results when these ingredients are sautéed on a low heat for several hours.

Tempeh: A traditional Indonesian soy food made from split soybeans, water, and special bacteria. Fermenting the soybeans for about one day can make tempeh, or it can be purchased ready-made in many natural food stores. High in protein and with a rich, appealing taste, tempeh is used in soups, stews, sandwiches, casseroles, and a variety of other dishes.

Tofu: Soybean curd made from soybeans processed with *nigari* (magnesium chloride, a component of salt).

Umeboshi Vinegar: Liquid that umeboshi plums are aged in. Also known as *ume-su*.

Wakame: A long, thin green sea vegetable used in making miso soup.

Whole Foods: Foods in their raw, unrefined, and unprocessed form, such as brown rice or whole quinoa. Also known as natural foods.

Whole Grains: Unrefined cereal grains to which nothing has been added or subtracted in milling except the inedible outer hull.

Wild Rice: A wild cereal grass native to North America.

Yang: One of the two fundamental energies of the universe. Yang refers to the relative tendency of contraction, centripetal force, density, heat, light, and other qualities. Yang energy tends to go down and inward in the vegetable kingdom. Yang predominates in small compact grains such as brown rice, millet, and buckwheat; in root vegetables; and in sea salt, miso, and tamari. Its complementary and antagonistic energy is yin.

Yin: One of the two fundamental energies of the universe. Yin refers to the relative tendency of expansion, growth, centrifugal force, diffusion, cold, darkness, and other qualities. Yin energy tends to go up and outward in the vegetable kingdom. Yin energy predominates in large whole grains (such as corn, oats, and barley), leafy green vegetables, oils, nuts, fruits, and most liquids. Its complementary and antagonistic energy is yang.

Acknowledgements

A heartfelt thanks to everyone who gave support to make this book a reality! Limited space allows us to mention only a few of you, but you know who you are.

Our deepest gratitude for seeding the modern macrobiotic teachings goes to the late George and Lima Ohsawa. We also wish to take this opportunity to extend worldwide a heartfelt note of thanks to the many macrobiotic teachers, authors, communities, practitioners, and businesses for their continued furtherance of this macrobiotic peaceful way of life.

A sincere appreciation goes to our extended families, children, and grandchildren, with special thanks to Midori Kushi, to Anne Leinen (for her cover design brain-storming), to Angelica Kushi and to her father Lawrence Haruo Kushi, PhD (son of Michio and Aveline Kushi) for his scientific input, and to the late Aveline Kushi for teaching the art of macrobiotic cooking.

A special thank you goes to the German editor, Richard Theobald, who supported this book idea from the start, and the Ost West Verlag (East West Publishing House). We also extend gratitude to the English editors Pat Samples, and especially to Lynn Cross for her diligent efforts to help us finish this project.

Much gratitude and thanks goes to the recipe testers, prop lenders, supporters, and friends: Laurie Savran, Anita Demants, Jim Bottomley of Red Eye Ceramics, Deborah Savran, Allison Widboom, Debbie Johnson, Anna Merle, Cheryl Locke, Kathleen Schuler, and Leslie Frodema. A special thank you goes to Gabriele's makeup artist and stylist, Cindy Rae, and the food and prop stylist par excellence, Jody Ann Lichtor and Susan Barrientos.

Thank you to the chefs who lent their wonderful recipes: Marie Digatono of Eco Yards & Gardens for *Dinosaur Kale Chips*; AmyLeo Barankovich of Vegan Affairs and Teaching Compassion for *Smoky Black-Peppered Seared Green Beans*; Michelle Licata, of Olives and Pearls Creative Organic Foods for *Tree Bean Salad*; Dawn Pallavi Ludwig, former owner of the Natural Epicurean Academy of Culinary Arts in Austin, Texas, for *Gluten-Free Crepes*; Gary Alinder, blogger and chef for 20+ years at the Monday Night Macrobiotic Dinners in Palo Alto, California, for *Gluten-Free Raspberry Cookie*; and Anne-Marie Fryer Wiboltt, author of *Cooking For the Love of The World*, for *Nettle Tea*.

We cannot thank enough photographer Allen Brown (a godsend) who made many of the recipes so visually enjoyable.

About the Authors

Gabriele Kushi

Gabriele Kushi, BFA, MEA, CHC, AADP studied alternative forms of nutrition and education at the Institute for Integrative Nutrition in conjunction with Columbia University, the Kushi Institute, and the University of Minnesota. She is an internationally known author, lecturer, health consultant and cooking teacher. Gabriele has dedicated her life to the healing arts, with special focus on the macrobiotic one peaceful world tradition, indigenous and alternative healing, the yogic sciences, sustainability, and the support of these arts by sound research.

She is the founder and director of Kushi's Kitchen (www.KushisKitchen.com), the author of *Embracing Menopause Naturally* (Square One Publishers, 2006), and the lecturer and cooking teacher of a *Macrobiotic Natural Foods Cooking DVD Series* that accompany *The Macrobiotic Kitchen in Ten Easy Steps* and her personal long-distance counseling and coaching programs.

Gabriele is often featured on radio talk shows and is widely quoted in print and electronic media. She has been published in the magazines *Natural Health, Taste for Life, Essential Wellness,* and in the seasonal publication *Das Grosse Leben* in Germany, among others.

She is a 1979 graduate of the Kushi Institute USA, and a Kushi Institute-certified macrobiotic teacher and counselor (MEA). She studied the universal macrobiotic yin and yang principles, the 5-energy transformation theory, whole foods cooking and healing with foods, health evaluation and counseling, as well as palm healing, shiatsu, and Do-In, with the Institute's founders, international macrobiotic leaders Aveline and Michio Kushi. Gabriele became a US-board-certified Holistic Health Practitioner in 2008 after studies at the Institute for Integrative Nutrition in conjunction with Columbia University Teachers College, New York City. She also holds a Bachelor of Fine Arts, summa cum laude degree in photography and Native American studies from the University of Minnesota.

Gabriele received the 2009 Aveline Kushi award for her dedication and work in macrobiotics, and served at the board of directors of Earth Save International. She also embraces the Native American medicine ways (since 1986) and collaborates with healers and spiritual leaders worldwide. Gabriele has traveled in Europe, Japan, Mexico, Middle America, India, the United States, and Africa.

Gabriele was born in Germany and lives for decades in the United States and has a daughter, Angelica Kushi. Michio and Aveline Kushi are her in-laws. Learn more at www.kushiskitchen.com

Michio Kushi

Michio Kushi was born in 1926 into a family of educators in Japan. During World War II, he studied political science and international law at Tokyo University. The atomic bombing of Hiroshima and Nagasaki made a deep impression on him, and he decided to devote his life to the pursuit of world peace. Kushi also studied in Japan with George Ohsawa, who taught that food was the key to health and that health was the key to peace. Ohsawa believed that humanity, by returning to a traditional diet of whole, natural foods, and living in harmony with one's environment would regain physical and mental balance and become more peaceful.

After the war, Kushi came to the United States to further his studies in political science as an avenue to world peace at Columbia University. However, he decided that he could make greater progress toward world peace by influencing individual consciousness through better food and personal health.

In 1966 Michio Kushi and his wife Aveline founded Erewhon the nation's pioneer natural foods distributor to make organically grown whole and naturally processed foods widely available, through sourcing of such grains and beans directly from farmers. Erewhon pioneered markets for artisanal products such as miso or shoyu that were made using traditional methods.

In 1969, his students founded East West Journal, initially a macrobiotic community newsletter that would grow into one of the first monthly magazines of the "new age" and alternative consciousness movements that grew out of the cultural upheavals of the 1960's. In 1972, the Kushi's founded the East West Foundation, established to spread macrobiotic education and research. In 1978 they founded the Kushi Institute, an educational organization for the training of future leaders of society, including macrobiotic teachers, counselors, and cooks. Students of the Kushi Institute and its affiliates in Amsterdam, London, and Tokyo, have gone on to become leaders of the natural foods, alternative health and macrobiotic communities in communities throughout the world. Kushi's worldwide seminars and lectures on the relationship of diet to degenerative disease and the reconstruction of modern humanity have attracted thousands of doctors, nurses, nutritionists, and other health-care professionals.

Over the years, the Kushi's life and teachings have been profiled in *The Boston Globe Magazine, Life, The Saturday Evening Post, Paris Match, Interview,* and many other publications. Kushi has written several dozen books, including *The Book of Macrobiotics, The Cancer Prevention Diet, Diet for a Strong Heart, One Peaceful World,* and *AIDS, Macrobiotics, and Natural Immunity.* In recognition of his role in launching macrobiotics and the modern health and diet revolution, the Smithsonian Institution established the "Michio and Aveline Kushi Collection, 1960-1997" of documents, materials, and artifacts associated with his life and times. For their "extraordinary contribution to diet, health, and world peace, and for serving as powerful examples of conscious living," Mr. and Mrs. Kushi were awarded the Peace Abbey Courage of Conscience Award in 2000. He has five children, thirteen grandchildren and two great-grandchildren.

Endnotes

[1] Christoph Wilhelm Hufeland, *Makrobiotik; Die Kunst, das menschliche Leben zu verlängern* (Germany, 1842).

[2] Ronald E. Kotzsch, Ph.D., *Macrobiotics Yesterday and Today.* Tokyo: Japan Publications, 1985.

[3] Michio Kushi. *The Book of Macrobiotics: The Universal Way of Health and Happiness,* Tokyo: Japan Publications, 1977.

[4] Aveline Kushi, with Alex Jack. *Aveline Kushi's Complete Guide to Macrobiotic Cooking for Health, Harmony, and Peace.* New York: Warner Books, 1988.

[5] Cornellia Aihara. *The Chico-San Cookbook: A Unique Guidebook to Natural Foods Cooking.* Chico, CA: Chico-San, 1972.

[6] Aveline Kushi, with Alex Jack. *Aveline: The Life and Dream Of The Woman Behind Macrobiotics Today.* New York: Japan Publications, 1988.

[7] Congressional Record, V. 145, Pt. 8, May 24, 1999 to June 8 1999.
http://web.ebscohost.com/ehost/detail?vid=5&sid=16e9ed64-7774-4649-9dce-ffd8e60ebe9e%40sessionmgr112&hid=121&bdata=JmF1dGh0eXBlPWdlbyZnZW9jdXN0aWQ9czM2MTM5MDQmc2l0ZT1laG9zdC1saXZl#db=awh&AN=9805241

[8] Dirk Benedict. *Confessions of a Kamikaze Cowboy.* New York: Square One Publishing, 2005.

[9] William Dufty. *Sugar Blues.* New York: Warner Books, 1976.

[10] Verne Varona. *Nature's Cancer-Fighting Foods,* Perigee, 2013, 14th edition; and *Macrobiotics For Dummies.* New York: Wiley Publishing, 2009.

[11] A. Sparber, et al., "Use of Complementary Medicine by Adult Patients Participating in Cancer Clinical Trials," *Oncology Nursing Forum* 27(4) (2000): 623–30.

[12] Jean Kohler and Mary Alice Kohler. *Healing Miracles from Macrobiotics: A Diet for All Seasons.* New York: Parker, 1979. [Recovery from terminal pancreatic cancer]

[13] Elaine Nussbaum. *Recovery: From Cancer to Health Through Macrobiotics.* New York: Japan Publications, 1986.
[14] Virginia Brown and Susan Stayman. *Macrobiotic Miracle: How a Vermont Family Overcame Cancer.* Tokyo: Japan Publications, 1984. [Recovery from malignant melanoma, Stage IV]

[15] Anthony J. Sattilaro, M.D. *Recalled By Life: The Story of My Recovery from Cancer,* Avon Books (MM) 1982.

16 Ann Fawcett and Cynthia Smith, compilers. *Cancer-Free: 30 Who Triumphed over Cancer Naturally,* New York: Japan Publications, 1991. [account of Kit Kitatani, a United Nations administrator from Japan who had untreatable stomach cancer]

17 Michio Kushi and Alex Jack. *The Cancer Prevention Diet*, New York: St. Martin's Press, 1994.

18 Michio Kushi. *The Do-In Way*, New York: Square One Publishing, 2006.

19 R. Mitchell. Is Physical Activity in Natural Environments Better for Mental Health than Physical Activity in Other Environments? *Social Science and Medicine, 91* (2013): 130-134. ISSN 0277-9536 (doi:10.1016/j.socscimed.2012.04.012)

20 *Harvard School of Public Health Newsletter, The Nutrition Source.* "Calcium and Milk," http://www.hsph.harvard.edu/nutritionsource/what-should-you-eat/calcium-and-milk/index.html

21 Y. Park et al., "Fruit and Vegetable Intakes and Risk of Colorectal Cancer in the NIH–AARP Diet and Health Study," *American Journal of Epidemiology 166(2)* (2007): 170-80.

22 "Milchkonsum: Sonderweg der Europäer," *Das Grosse Leben Makrobiotik-Magazine* 82 (2010): 18-21.
["Milk Consumption: 'Special Path' of the Europeans," *The Great Life Macrobiotic Magazine 82* (2010): 18-21.]

23 *Harvard School of Public Health Newsletter*, "Calcium and Milk."

24 *Harvard School of Public Health Newsletter*, "Healthy Eating Plate and Healthy Eating Pyramid."

25 Elena Conis, "Ancient Grains, the Best Thing Since Sliced Bread?" *Los Angeles Times*, February 19, 2011.

26 Thompson, Tricia, and Marlisa Brown. *American Dietetic Association Easy Gluten-Free: Expert Nutrition Advice with More than 100 Recipes.* Hoboken, NJ: John Wiley & Sons, 2010/2014.
27 Paul Pitchford, *Healing with Whole Foods: Asian Traditions and Modern Nutrition,* 3rd edition. Berkeley, CA: North Atlantic Books, 2002, 492.

28 J. M. Kawa, C. G. Taylor, and R. Przybylski, "Buckwheat Concentrate Reduces Serum Glucose in Streptozotocin-diabetic Rats," *Journal of Agricultural and Food Chemistry, 51* (2003).

29 J. F. Ludvigsson, et al., "Small-intestinal Histopathology and Mortality Risk in Celiac Disease," *Journal of the American Medical Association 302*(11) (2009): 1171-8.

30 United States Food and Drug Administration, "Additional Information on Acrylamide, Diet, and Food Storage and Preparation" (May 22, 2008).

31 Panel on Macronutrients, Institute of Medicine of the National Academies, *Dietary Reference Intakes for Energy, Carbohydrate, Fiber, Fat, Fatty Acids, Cholesterol, Protein, and Amino Acids*, Washington, DC: National Academies Press, 2005.

[32] V. R. Young and P. L. Pellett, "Plant Proteins in Relation to Human Protein and Amino Acid Nutrition," *American Journal of Clinical Nutrition 59* (suppl) (1994): 1203S-1212S.

[33] A. R. Mangels, V. Messina, and V. Melina, "Position of The American Dietetic Association and Dietitians of Canada: Vegetarian Diets," *Journal of the American Dietetic Association 103*(6) (2003): 748-65.

[34] Ken Albala, *Beans: A History*, Google eBook, 2007.

[35] Frances M. Lappe, *Diet for a Small Planet*, New York: Ballantine Books, 1991.

[36] Frances M. Lappe and Anna Lappe, *Hope's Edge, the Next Diet for a Small Planet,* New York: Tarcher, 2003.

[37] T. C. Campbell and T. M. Campbell, *The China Study,* Dallas, TX: BenBella Books, 2005.

[38] Debra Wasserman and Reed Mangels, *Simply Vegan: Quick Vegetarian Meals,* Baltimore, MD: Vegetarian Resource Group, 2006.

[39] World Cancer Research Fund/American Institute for Cancer Research, *Food, Nutrition and the Prevention of Cancer: A Global Perspective,* Washington, DC: WCRF/AICR, 1997.

[40] Dean Ornish et al., "Can Lifestyle Changes Reverse Coronary Heart Disease?" *The Lancet 336* (1990): 129-133.

[41] "Position of the American Dietetic Association, Dietitians of Canada, and the American College of Sports Medicine: Nutrition and Athletic Performance," *Journal of the American Dietetic Association 100* (2000): 1543-56.

[42] W. Zheng et al., "The Shanghai Women's Health Study: Rationale, Study Design, and Baseline Characteristics," *American Journal of Epidemiology 162*(11) (2005): 1123-31.

[43] Gabriele Kushi, *Embracing Menopause Naturally,* New York: Square One Publishers, 2006.

[44] M. Messina and C. Hughes, "Efficacy of Soy Foods and Soybean Isoflavone Supplements for Alleviating Menopausal Symptoms Is Positively Related to Initial Hot Flash Frequency," *Journal of Medicinal Food 6* (2003): 1-11.

[45] D. Zohary and M. Hopf, *Domestication of Plants in the Old World,* 3rd ed., New York: Oxford University Press, 2000.

[46] Kay Fleming, "Timpsula, Turnip of the Prairie," Manataka American Indian Council, Smoke *Signal Newsletter* VII (2005).

[47] Pliny the Elder, *The Natural History.* Translated by John Bostock, M. D. and H. T. Riley, London: Taylor and Francis, 1855.

[48] Linda Stradley, "Daikon Radish." http://whatscookingamerica.net/DaikonRadish.htm

[49] Klaire Brown, "The History of Butternut Squash." http://www.ehow.com/facts_7258933_history-butternut-squash.html

[50] University of Saskatchewan College of Agriculture and Bioresources, "The History of Cabbage." http://agbio.usask.ca/veg-cabbage

[51] David Heber, M.D., *What Color Is Your Diet?* New York: HarperCollins, 2002.

[52] Katz, Sandor Ellix, *The Art of Fermentation*, Vermont: Chelsea Green Publishing, 2012.

[53] Michio Kushi and Alex Jack, *One Peaceful World: Michio Kushi's Approach To Creating A Healthy And Harmonious Mind, Home, And World Community*, New York: St. Martin's Press, 1987.

[54] M. Indergaard and J. Minsaas, "Animal and Human Nutrition," in *Seaweed Resources in Europe: Uses and Potential,* ed. M. D. Guiry and G. Blunden, Hoboken, NJ: John Wiley & Sons, 1991.

[55] Isabella Abbott, "The Uses of Seaweed as Food in Hawaii," *Economic Botany 32*(4): 409-412.

[56] R. Elkins, *Limu Moui: Prize Sea Plant of Tonga And the South Pacific*, Salt Lake City, UT: Woodland Publishing, 2001.

[57] S. V. Hallsson, "The Uses of Seaweed in Iceland," *Proceedings of the Fourth International Seaweed Symposium* (France, 1961).

[58] C. K. Tseng, "Marine Phycoculture in China," *Proceedings of the International Seaweed Symposium 10* (1981): 124-152.

[59] Dennis J. McHugh, *A Guide to the Seaweed Industry. FAO Fisheries Technical Paper 441*, Rome: Food and Agriculture Organization of the United Nations, 2003.

[60] M. E. Mitchell and M. D. Guiry, "Carrageen: A Local Habitation or a Name?" *Journal of Ethnopharmacology 9* (1983): 347-51.

[61] Weston Price, D.D.S., *Nutrition and Physical Degeneration,* New Canaan, CT: Keats Publishing, 1997.

[62] Y. D. Tanaka, D. Waldron-Edward, and S. C. Skoryna, "Studies on Inhibition of Intestinal Absorption of Radioactive Strontium. VII. Relationship of Biological Activity to Chemical Composition of Alginates Obtained from North American Seaweeds," *Canadian Medical Association Journal 99*(4) (1968): 169-75.

[63] Y. F. Gong et al., "Suppression of Radioactive Strontium Absorption by Sodium Alginate in Animals and Human Subjects," *Biomedical and Environmental Sciences, 4*(3) (1991): 273-82.

[64] R. Gupta et al., "Microbial Biosorbents: Meeting Challenges of Heavy Metal Pollution in Aqueous Solutions, *Current Science 78* (2000): 967-973.

[65] T. A. Davis, B. Volesky, and A. Mucci, "A Review of the Biochemistry of Heavy Metal Biosorption by Brown Algae," *Water Research 37* (2003): 4311-30.

[66] K. Lau et al., "Synergistic Interactions Between Commonly Used Food additives in a Developmental Neurotoxicity Test," *Toxicological Sciences 90*(1) (2006): 178-87.

[67] I. Yamamoto et al., "Antitumor Effect of Seaweeds," *Japanese Journal of Experimental Medicine* 44 (1974): 543-46.

[68] J. Teas, "The Dietary Intake of Laminaria, a Brown Seaweed, and Breast Cancer Prevention," *Nutrition and Cancer* 4(3) (1983): 217-22.

[69] J. Teas, J. et al., "Seaweed and Soy: Companion Foods in Asian Cuisine and Their Effects on Thyroid Function in American Women," *Journal of Medicinal Food* 10 (2007): 90-100.

[70] F. Watanabe et al., "Characterization of a Vitamin B12 Compound in the Edible Purple Laver, Porphyra Yezoensis, *Bioscience, Biotechnology, and Biochemistry* 64(12) (2000): 2712-5.

[71] P. Dagnelie, W. A. van Staveren, and H. van den Berg, "Vitamin B-12 from Algae Appears Not to Be Bioavailable," *American Journal of Clinical Nutrition* 53 (1991): 695-7.

[72] M. Indergaard and J. Minsaas, "Animal and Human Nutrition," in *Seaweed Resources in Europe: Uses and Potential,* ed. M. D. Guiry and G. Blunden, Hoboken, NJ: John Wiley & Sons, 1991.

[73] Karl J. Abrams, *Algae to the Rescue! Everything You Need to Know About Nutritional Blue-Green Algae,* Wayne City, NE: Logan House, 1996.

[74] Karl J. Abrams, *Attention Deficit Hyperactivity Disorder: A Nutritional Approach,* Chelsea, MI: Timeless Books Publications, 1998.

[75] Fereydoon Batmanghelidj, *Your Body's Many Cries for Water*, Falls Church, VA: Global Health Solutions, 2008.

[76] Theodore A. Baroody, *Alkalize or Die: Superior Health Through Proper Alkaline-Acid Balance,* Waynesville, NC: Eclectic Press, 1996.

[77] Diane Gow McDilda, *The Everything Green Living Book: Easy Ways to Conserve Energy, Protect Your Family's Health, and Help Save the Environment,* Avon, MA: Adams Media Corporation, 2007.

[78] Nieca Goldberg, M.D., *The Women's Healthy Heart Program: Lifesaving Strategies for Preventing and Healing Heart Disease*, New York: Ballantine Books, 2006.

[79] Rodney J. Green et al., "Common Tea Formulations Modulate In Vitro Digestive Recovery of Green Tea Catechins," *Molecular Nutrition & Food Research* 51(9) (2007): 1152-62.

[80] B. A. Cassady et al., "Mastication of Almonds: Effects of Lipid Bioaccessibility, Appetite, and Hormone Response," *American Journal of Clinical Nutrition* 89(3) (2009): 794-800.

[81] Masaru Emoto, *The Miracle of Water*, New York: Atria Books, 2011.

[82] June Crosby and Ruth Conrad Bateman, *Serve It Cold! A Cookbook of Delicious Cold Dishes*, New York: Gramercy Publishing Company, 1968.

[83] Jonathan R. Schultes, Production. North Carolina Cooperative Extension Service, North Carolina State University. Revised 12/94.

[84] J. Paniagua, et al., "A MUFA-rich Diet Improves Postprandial Glucose, Lipid and GLP-1 Responses in Insulin-resistant Subjects," *Journal of the American College of Nutrition 26* (2007): 434.

[85] J. Paniagua, et al., "A MUFA-rich Diet Improves Postprandial Glucose, Lipid and GLP-1 Responses in Insulin-resistant Subjects," *Journal of the American College of Nutrition 26* (2007): 434.

[86] P. Angerer and C. von Schacky, "n-3 Polyunsaturated Fatty Acids and the Cardiovascular System," *Current Opinion in Lipidology 11*(1) (2000): 57-63.

[87] B. Bahadori, et al., "Omega-3 Fatty Acids Infusions as Adjuvant Therapy in Rheumatoid Arthritis," *Journal of Parenteral and Enteral Nutrition 34(2)* (2010): 151-5.

[88] A. Aben and M. Danckaerts, "Omega-3 and Omega-6 Fatty Acids in the Treatment of Children and Adolescents with ADHD," *Tijdschrift Voor Psychiatry 52(2)* (2010): 89-97.

[89] I. A. Brouwer, et al., "Dietary -Linolenic Acid Is Associated with Reduced Risk of Fatal Coronary Heart Disease, but Increased Prostate Cancer Risk: A Meta-Analysis," *Journal of Nutrition 134*(4): 919-22.

[90] World Health Organization, "Diet, Nutrition, and the Prevention of Chronic Diseases," *WHO Technical Report Series 916* (2003): 81-94.

[91] EFSA Panel on Dietetic Products, Nutrition, and Allergies (NDA), "Scientific Opinion on Dietary Reference Values for Fats, Including Saturated Fatty Acids, Polyunsaturated Fatty Acids, Monounsaturated Fatty Acids, Trans Fatty Acids, and Cholesterol," *EFSA Journal 8*(3), (2010): 1461. DOI: 10.2903/j.efsa.2010.1461

[92] M. A. Flynn, et al., "Serum Lipids and Eggs," *Journal of the American Dietetic Association 86*(11) (1986): 1541-8.

[93] S. M. Teegala, et al., "Consumption and Health Effects of Trans Fatty Acids: A Review," *Journal of AOAC International 92* (2009): 1250.

[94] J. Ruano, et al., "Phenolic Content of Virgin Olive Oil Improves Ischemic Reactive Hyperemia in Hypercholesterolemic Patients," *Journal of the American College of Cardiology 46*(10) (2005): 1864-8.

[95] G. K. Beauchamp, et al., "Anti-inflammatory Effect of Virgin Olive Oil in Stable Coronary Disease Patients: A Randomized, Crossover, Controlled Trial," *European Journal of Clinical Nutrition 62* (2008): 570–574. DOI: 10.1038/sj.ejcn.1602724

[96] K. M. Phillips, et al., "Phytosterol Composition of Nuts and Seeds Commonly Consumed in the United States," *Journal of Agricultural and Food Chemistry 53(24)* (2005): 9436-45.

[97] Janice R. Herman, Ph.D., RD/LD., *Dietary Sugar and Alternative Sweeteners,* Stillwater, OK: Oklahoma Cooperative Extension Service, 1999.

[98] Other names are beet sugar, buttered syrup, cane juice crystals, cane sugar, caramel, carob syrup, date sugar, dextran, diastase, diastatic malt, ethyl maltol, evaporated cane juice, fruit juice or fruit juice concentrate, glucose, glucose solids, golden sugar, golden syrup, grape sugar, honey, invert sugar, lactose/milk sugar, malt syrup, maltodextrin, maltose, mannitol, maltitol,

molasses, raw sugar, refiner's syrup, stevia, sorbitol, sorghum syrup, sucrose or table sugar, sugar, turbinado sugar, yellow sugar, jaggery.

[99] Melanie Warner, "The Lowdown on Sweet?" *The New York Times*, February 12, 2006.

[100] Annemarie Colbin, PhD, "Aspartame, The Real Story." http://www.foodandhealing.com/articles/article-aspartame.htm

[101] Connie Bennett and Stephen Sinatra, *Sugar Shock!* New York: Berkley Books, 2006.

[102] Michio Kushi, *The Macrobiotic Way of Natural Healing*, Boston: East West Publications, 1978.

[103] William Dufty, *Sugar Blues*, New York: Warner Books, 1976.

[104] Nicole M. Avena, Pedro Rada, and Bartley G. Hoebel, "Sugar and Fat Bingeing Have Notable Differences in Addictive-like Behavior," *The Journal of Nutrition 139*(3) (2009): 623-8.

[105] Nancy Appleton, PhD, *Lick The Sugar Habit*, New York: Warner Books, 1986.

[106] Annemarie Colbin, PhD, *The Whole-Food Guide to Strong Bones: A Holistic Approach*, Oakland, CA: New Harbinger Publications, 2009.

[107] L. Cohen, L. G. Curhan, and J. Forman, "Association of Sweetened Beverage Intake with Incident Hypertension," *Journal of General Internal Medicine 27*(9) (2012): 1127-34.

[108] World Cancer Research Fund/American Institute for Cancer Research, *Food, Nutrition and the Prevention of Cancer: A Global Perspective,* Washington, DC: WCRF/AICR, 1997.

[109] Nancy Appleton, *Lick the Sugar Habit,* New York: Avery, 1985.

[110] Anne-Marie Fryer Wiboltt, *Cooking for the Love of the World,* Goldenstone Press, 2008.

[111] Michio Kushi, *The Do-In Way: Gentle Exercises to Liberate the Body, Mind, and Spirit*, New York: Square One Publishing, 2006.

[112] Visit the Isha Yoga Foundation website for further instructions.

Recipe Index

CPSIA information can be obtained
at www.ICGtesting.com
Printed in the USA
FSOW03n1019170616
21687FS

9 783930 564408